withdraws wc H

Pain: Causes and Management

Jan Hawthorn, BSc, PhD
&
Kathy Redmond, MSc, RGN

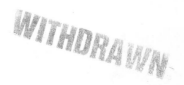

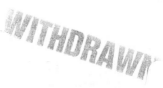

**Blackwell
Science**

© Jan Hawthorn and Kathy Redmond 1998

Blackwell Science Ltd
Editorial Offices:
Osney Mead, Oxford OX2 0EL
25 John Street, London WC1N 2BL
23 Ainslie Place, Edinburgh EH3 6AJ
350 Main Street, Malden
  MA 02148 5018, USA
54 University Street, Carlton
  Victoria 3053, Australia
10, rue Casimir Delavigne
  75006 Paris, France

Other Editorial Offices:

Blackwell Wissenschafts-Verlag GmbH
Kurfürstendamm 57
10707 Berlin, Germany

Blackwell Science KK
MG Kodenmacho Building
7-10 Kodenmacho Nihombashi
Chuo-ku, Tokyo 104, Japan

The right of the Author to be identified as
the Author of this Work has been asserted in
accordance with the Copyright, Designs and
Patents Act 1988.

All rights reserved. No part of this
publication may be reproduced, stored in a
retrieval system, or transmitted, in any form
or by any means, electronic, mechanical,
photocopying, recording or otherwise,
except as permitted by the UK Copyright,
Designs and Patents Act1988, without the
prior permission of the copyright owner.

First published 1998

Reprinted 1999

Set in 10/12pt Sabon
by DP Photosetting, Aylesbury, Bucks.
Printed and bound in Great Britain by
Biddles Ltd, Guildford and King's Lynn

The Blackwell Science logo is a trade mark
of Blackwell Science Ltd, registered at the
United Kingdom Trade Marks Registry

DISTRIBUTORS

Marston Book Services Ltd
PO Box 269
Abingdon
Oxon OX14 4YN
(*Orders:* Tel: 01235 465500
        Fax: 01235 465555)

USA
Blackwell Science, Inc.
Commerce Place
350 Main Street
Malden, MA 02148 5018
(*Orders:* Tel: 800 759 6102
             781 388 8250
        Fax: 781 388 8255)

Canada
Login Brothers Book Company
324 Saulteaux Crescent
Winnipeg, Manitoba R3J 3T2
(*Orders:* Tel: 204 837 2987
        Fax: 204 837 3116)

Australia
Blackwell Science Pty Ltd.
54 University Street
Carlton, Victoria 3053
(*Orders:* Tel: 03 9347 0300
        Fax: 03 9347 5001)

A catalogue record for this title
is available from the British Library

ISBN 0-632-04033-5

Library of Congress
Cataloging-in-Publication Data
Hawthorn, Jan.
    Pain: causes and management/
    Jan Hawthorn & Kathy Redmond.
       p. cm.
    Includes bibliographical references
    and index.
    ISBN 0-632-04033-5 (pbk.)
    1. Pain-Nursing. 2. Chronic pain
    - Nursing. 3. Pain - Treatment.
    4. Chronic pain - Treatment.
    I. Redmond, Kathy. II. Title.
    [DNLM: 1. Pain - etiology. 2. Pain -
    nursing. 3. Nursing Process.
    WL704 H399p 1998]
    RB127.H39 1998
    616'.0472 - dc21
    DNLM/DLC
    for Library of Congress   98-25009
                                       CIP

For further information on
Blackwell Science, visit our website:
www.blackwell-science.com

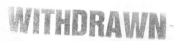

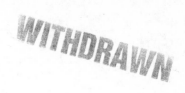

Contents

WITHDRAWN

To Sophie and Alberto

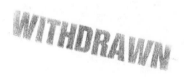

Acknowledgements

We are indebted to Dr Martin Perkins for his comments on the physiology of pain, and to Dr John Henderson for numerous contributions and invaluable discussions, and for drawing the illustration on page 11.

Chapter 1

Introduction

Pain is a universal experience that can span an enormous spectrum of intensity from mild discomfort to excruciating agony. The term pain can also denote a variety of feelings. Readers are likely to think first of pain as the physical sensation associated with tissue damage or disease, but the term can also denote various emotions: 'a painful experience'; 'a painful loss'; 'a pain-in-the-neck'; 'she's a real pain'. Pain may not only have a physical dimension; it often has an emotional and spiritual component, and each aspect deserves attention if pain is to be ameliorated successfully.

Pain is a subjective experience and is, therefore, unique to each individual. Each person's experience of pain is different; and it is important to remember that, given the same set of circumstances, the pain felt will differ markedly from person to person. This is perhaps one of the most fundamental aspects of pain management that must be borne in mind by anyone caring for patients in pain. The underlying cause of the pain will not predict how much pain is experienced by any one person. Each individual has a different ability to tolerate pain and a different approach to being able to cope with the pain, and similarly each individual will respond in their own way to any treatment offered for pain relief.

The emotional aspect of pain will vary considerably with each individual; and an overriding influence will be the nature and severity of the disease, or the underlying cause of the pain and whether the pain has an identifiable source. The discomfort of a new mother who has recently delivered a perfect baby cannot be compared to the pain of a woman who has experienced a stillbirth; a terminally ill cancer patient will have a very different view of pain to the those in whom the disease is operable and the prognosis hopeful.

So, while the ground rules of good nursing care – that is: determining causes, identifying appropriate interventions, giving suitable treatment, and monitoring the success of that treatment – will always apply, the nurse caring for a patient in pain must always remember that good communication and interaction with that person is crucial to effective pain management.

How do we talk about pain? Most of the vocabulary of pain relies on past experience: 'It felt as sharp as a needle', 'It was a burning pain', 'A stabbing pain', 'A throbbing pain'. How can we relate to these descriptions if we have never felt a needle, a burn, a stab, a throbbing? Even the International Association for the Study of Pain (Anon, 1979) says in its definition, 'Pain is a subjective experience. Each individual learns the application of the word through experiences related to injury in early life'. So pain is universal and we rely on previous experience to allow us to communicate our subjective feelings. Sometimes it is impossible for the patient to convey the reality of his or her pain experience.

1.1 The role of pain

The vocabulary of pain always suggests a negative event – an unpleasant experience. But, if pain is so much a part of daily life, does it perhaps have a positive role? In basic biological terms pain is indeed a protective mechanism. If you place your hand on something that is very hot, then you will withdraw your hand instantaneously, almost before there is conscious perception of the pain. The sharp, burning sensation has caused you to remove your hand from the source of further injury. To look in purely biological terms we must imagine animals – perhaps our ancestors – for them this kind of pain needs to be instant, intense and short lived. It signals a dangerous situation to the animal involved, and the animal may need to be able to run away from the danger. Such pain is also a learning experience, so the young animal will learn to avoid that particular source of danger in the future.

Later, a duller, more persistent pain may ensue. This pain will ensure that you use your hand carefully, protecting it from further abuse and allowing a period of healing to occur. For animals the duller, slow pain may well be accompanied by feelings of wretchedness or misery which causes them to find a safe, protected place to rest so that healing can occur.

Dull aching pains can also signal that something is wrong, such as a strained joint or an infection. Again this may signal to the animal that it needs to rest and allow healing to occur. For man (and his domesticated animals) medical or veterinary assistance can be sought.

However, this teleological argument is clearly not the whole story, as there are several instances where pain serves no useful purpose or where pain comes too late to be helpful. There are also instances of spontaneously occurring pain that have no (apparently) identifiable cause.

For example, patients who have had a limb amputated will often still feel pain in the amputated limb. This pain is not only distressing but does not benefit the individual in any obvious way. The pain becomes a medical condition, by contrast to a symptom of an underlying condition, and the pain, not the disease, needs treatment. Even though we may be able to explain physiologically why this happens, such pain is not only unhelpful, having no obvious positive role, but also can be considered as detrimental.

Pain after surgery is, while perhaps understandable, detrimental to healing. It causes patients to resist recovering mobility, which brings complications such as deep vein thrombosis (DVT) and chest infection, and can cause depression and loss of morale.

Pain can be responsible for decreased food intake and impaired sleep, thereby causing debility, poor response to treatment and delayed healing. Pain that does not resolve after the apparent cause of the pain has been treated can be especially depressing. Any pain will interfere with normal daily functioning, lowering quality of life; and constant intractable pain has been identified as a cause of suicide.

While pain signals danger, or something wrong, some diseases do not present with pain until the situation is way beyond salvage by medical intervention – e.g. ovarian cancer. At the other end of the spectrum is the condition of total lack of the sensation of pain. There are cases documented of individuals who were born without any pain sensation at all. These are described in detail in Melzack and Wall (1982). It is easy to see how small children without any pain sensations will soon injure themselves quite severely. Without the danger signal of pain they touch hot objects, cut themselves or suffer severe knocks. But the total lack of pain has more insidious ways of being detrimental. Undue stress may be placed on joints which become inflamed but this is not noticed without the warning signal of pain. Infections can become established beyond the reach of antibiotics if the infected tissue does not give out any messages. A total lack of pain is, therefore, a serious condition; and those reported in the literature have all resulted in the premature death of the individual – usually due to infections.

So the purpose of pain in multifactorial and some of its roles are more apparent than others. It is the negative aspects of pain that are usually encountered by nurses. A cardinal responsibility of nurses is to ensure that the best quality of life is maintained as much as possible for patients and that complications of pain are avoided; optimal pain management is crucial in realising this goal.

1.2 Perception and expression of pain

As we have said, pain is a subjective and a unique experience. Different individuals experiencing the same stimulus will perceive the pain differently, just as the same individual will have different experiences of pain in response to the same event on different occasions. These phenomena have given rise to the concept of a pain threshold – the level at which a stimulus is perceived as painful. There can be staggering variations in pain thresholds even within the same individual. Often quoted are reports by soldiers who, in the exhilaration and excitement of battle, suffered horrific wounds without feeling any pain. Yet, later in the calm of a hospital they flinched at the far less traumatic sensations of injections (Beecher, 1956). This is a real difference in threshold – the injury was not felt and may even have been unnoticed during the time of battle when the individual's threshold was high, but considerably less painful stimuli were uncomfortable when the individual's threshold was low. Threshold is the level at which pain is felt (this will be covered in more detail in Chapter 4).

Allied to threshold is tolerance to pain which is distinguished from threshold in that the individual is aware of the pain occurring but is prepared to bear it without displaying distress or seeking analgesic medication. A woman in labour may eschew analgesic medication out of concern for her baby, or a wish to undergo the experience of childbirth in a totally natural way. Under other circumstances, the same woman may not tolerate a far less painful toothache without reaching for the aspirin.

So threshold and tolerance are strongly influenced by circumstances as well as the individual's personality. Some factors that are influential are emotional state, sense of control, religious beliefs and gender. Upbringing and culture will also have effects on how people express their pain. Societies where public emotional displays are not acceptable are more likely to produce stoical individuals who do not readily admit to pain or seek assistance. Individuals coming from cultures where feelings are freely expressed may not be so reluctant to admit to pain or the need for analgesic intervention. Different individuals will have different problems in verbalising their pain (also discussed in greater detail in Chapter 4).

1.3 Incidence of pain

There is little information on the incidence of pain from all causes. Many studies have focused on cancer pain and suggest that moderate to severe cancer pain is experienced by about one-third of patients receiving active therapy, and by 56 to 90% of patients with advanced disease (Foley, 1979; Daut & Cleeland, 1982; Ahles *et al.*, 1984a). Pain is significantly greater with metastatic disease than with local or regional disease, and bone metastases seem to be the major cause of pain. It is conservatively estimated by the WHO that at least 4 million people are currently suffering from cancer pain with or without satisfactory analgesic treatment (Foley, 1993). However, in terms of both the number of patients suffering and, in many cases, the length of time the patient is in pain, cancer is overshadowed by the pain of chronic non-malignant disease. The list can never be comprehensive, but notable culprits for causing much misery are arthritic disease, neuropathies, peripheral vascular disease, shingles, AIDS, back pain, migraine, angina.

It is incredibly difficult to make any meaningful comparison between the incidence of different types of pain, since the methodology for pain measurement varies so widely. This variation is due to different criteria for defining pain and to the use of assessment tools that are specific for one type of pain but inappropriate for others. This can be illustrated by the study of chronic musculoskeletal pain (Magni *et al.*, 1993) which compared two surveys carried out by the United States Center for Health Statistics: one survey gave the incidence of persistent pain as 15%, the second survey carried out eight years later and using different criteria found the incidence to be 32.8%.

1.4 Undertreatment or inappropriate treatment of pain

Despite the universal nature of pain, it is sadly too often true that pain is not treated adequately. The undertreatment of pain was first reported in the early 1970s (Marks & Sachar, 1973) and has been noted by several authors in different clinical situations, most notably in cancer patients and post-surgically (Cohen, 1980; Kuhn *et al.*, 1990; McCaffery & Beebe, 1994; Melzack, 1990; Owen *et al.*, 1990).

Inadequacy of treatment of pain is due to a variety of factors including poor training of healthcare professionals in pain assessment and management, myths and misconceptions about pain and the use of opioids, and problems with the healthcare system. Pain assessment is a complicated process which can be hampered for a number of reasons including poor communication skills on the part of the healthcare professional, the values, attitudes and beliefs held by healthcare professionals, by patients and their families and finally as a result of the patients' reluctance or inability to express pain. This reluctance can be due to a fatalistic belief that pain is an inevitable consequence of their disease or to the fact that some patients do not want to be a nuisance or detract the doctor from treating their disease.

The achievement of effective pain relief is often compromised by inappropriate treatment goals; bizarre decisions surrounding the prescription and administration of analgesics and a reluctance to use complementary interventions, such as massage or the application of heat and cold. Bureaucratic procedures surrounding the administration of analgesics can exacerbate this problem. Patients also contribute to this problem by not taking prescribed analgesics. They do this because they often believe that analgesics should only be taken if absolutely necessary in order to have something available when things get really bad; they have concerns about unmanageable side effects, and some hold the belief that pain has a moral value that builds character. Sometimes, despite the best efforts of the clinical team, it is just not possible to provide constant, adequate pain relief; and the individual may need to be educated into coping with the presence of some degree of permanent pain (to be discussed in greater detail in Chapter 5).

However, it is worth discussing here that fear of taking medication features prominently in many patients' attitudes to pain. Of all analgesics the use of opioids is bedevilled by misconceptions and ill-founded fears –

the often called 'opio phobia'. Such misunderstandings occur on the part of healthcare professionals and patients alike. Where knowledge is poor, opioids may be associated with addiction. Doctors meter out doses of opioids sparingly, prescribing too low a dose or spacing the doses too far apart for adequate pain control, sometimes 'saving' them for when all else fails. Patients too associate opioids with drug addiction or think that if they are prescribed morphine, then their condition must be terminal. It is important that nurses, who are at the coal-face in pain control, understand these concerns and are able to elicit accurate assessments of pain from their patients.

1.5 The nurse's contribution to pain management

Nurses play a pivotal role in the management of pain. As discussed previously, pain is a multi-dimensional phenomenon. The onus is on the nurse to identify clearly the many factors which might be influencing the patient's perception and expression of pain. This may take some time to establish and the quality of the information collected is very much determined by the nurse's observational and interpersonal skills. Pain measurement tools can provide information which complements that collected through observation and interview and provides objective data about the patient's pain which is difficult for healthcare professionals to ignore.

Nurses bring enormous influence to bear on the choice of analgesic agent prescribed by doctors. Moreover, they make independent decisions regarding the timing, route of administration and the dose of drug administered. Nurses also play an important role in the prevention and management of the side effects of analgesic agents. To fulfil all of the above mentioned roles the nurse must have a thorough understanding of the action of analgesic agents, their side effects, dosages and frequency of use in different circumstances. A discussion on these issues is contained in a number of different chapters in this book, most notably in Chapters 6 and 7.

The multi-faceted nature of pain means that it is unlikely that pharmacological interventions will ameliorate it successfully in all situations. Therefore, a number of non-pharmacological interventions should be employed to complement the activity of analgesic agents. These interventions, which include a range of cognitive-behavioural strategies and cutaneous stimulation, are discussed in depth in Chapter 8. A discussion of the nurse's role in the provision of these interventions is contained in Chapter 6.

Chapter 2

The Physiology of Pain

Pain is a complex phenomenon which varies under different circumstances. This complexity is reflected in a certain plasticity (or fluidity) in the physiological processes mediating pain. Ideas at the beginning of the last century concentrated on the defensive component of acute pain and much of the research led to describing the pathways involved in the more straightforward, obvious pains such as a pinprick. This led to the erroneous belief that the peripheral mechanisms involved in all pain perception were understood. If pain perception were indeed this simple, then controlling pain in such a system would simply involve identifying the pathway and then interrupting the pain pathway at some point (McMahon & Koltzenburg, 1990).

However, we know that in the clinical situation pain is far more complex than this. It is not just a matter of the presence of stimuli which cause pain; but when disease, infection or trauma occur, some changes take place so that normal body functions and previously innocuous stimuli cause pain. In such situations pain may occur spontaneously or be evoked by innocent, everyday activities such as walking, coughing, moving and so on. Research in recent years has thrown more light on the complexity of pain perception and with more sophisticated techniques, we now know that many pain situations have a more subtle underlying physiology.

There are many ways of talking about pain, and selecting the most appropriate way of classifying pain will depend on the circumstances. For example, when trying to make a diagnosis of the cause of the pain we may be interested in whether it is somatic or visceral pain, but this classification is clearly of no use when talking to a patient! When eliciting information from a patient, it may be of more use to find out if the pain is constant or intermittent, whether it is sharp or dull and so on. These different ways of looking at pain will be described in more detail in Chapter 3, but it may be easier to understand these classifications if we first look at the underlying physiology of pain.

2.1 Physiological pain and pathological pain

To understand pain it must be recognised that in physiological terms there are two separate pain phenomena. The first is the pain that results from intense or potentially damaging stimuli (the pinprick). This pain, which is produced by stimulation of specialised pain-sensitive receptors (see below), is termed nociceptive or physiological pain. Nociceptive derives from the Latin *nocere* meaning 'to hurt'. Noxious, therefore, means hurtful or potentially damaging to tissue. The second type of pain occurs in pathological situations where changes occur in response to disease or trauma and low intensity or normally innocuous stimuli cause pain – termed pathological pain (Woolf, 1991). This usually follows nerve or tissue damage and is not a single entity – several different mechanisms underlie pathological pain. It is characterised by a disruption of normal mechanisms so that the pain occurs in the absence of an obvious stimulus, in response to innocuous stimuli, and in a prolonged or exaggerated fashion to noxious stimuli.

Physiological pain

Pain is a subjective phenomenon. The perception and interpretation of an event as being painful depends on higher brain centres – in other words, 'pain' as such does not exist unless and until it is interpreted by the central nervous system (CNS). Processes occurring in the periphery do not by themselves constitute pain. For this reason it is preferable to use the terms 'nociceptive pathways' and 'nociceptive receptors' rather than 'pain pathways' or 'pain receptors'.

Receptors are the specialised part of a cell, usually, but not always, on the cell surface, that recognise specialised substances that are delivering messages from other cells. Messengers may be neuro-transmitters, hormones, inflammatory mediators, etc.

The processes of perception and response to pain may be summarised as four phases:

- transduction – when the stimulus is detected by nociceptive receptors;
- transmission – when the message is relayed from the receptors to the central nervous system (CNS);
- modulation – when the message is modified by other activity in the body, which may be activity of other peripheral nerves or may occur in the CNS;
- perception – when the brain perceives the sensation as painful.

Nociceptive receptors

Nociceptive receptors are free nerve endings that are widely distributed throughout the body. There are three basic types of nociceptive receptors: chemical receptors, mechanical receptors and thermal receptors.

- Chemical receptors can be stimulated by external chemicals – examples are the sting of a wasp or a nettle – but the body's own chemicals can also irritate these receptors. Thus when tissue is cut or burned or a cell is ruptured by excessive pressure, a variety of chemicals are released. These include agents such as 5-hydroxytryptamine (5-HT or serotonin), histamine, potassium ions (K^+) or acetylcholine. Damage can also cause other inflammatory mediators to be synthesised such as bradykinin or cytokines.
- Mechanical receptors can respond to direct mechanical pressure such as squeezing or crushing, or to the pressure occurring as a consequence of tissue inflammation or oedema.
- Thermal receptors respond to extremes of heat or cold.

Receptors have a defined area from which they receive information. This is termed their receptive field. These free nerve endings respond to noxious stimuli and transmit this information via afferent, or sensory, fibres to the CNS. Primary afferent nociceptors are sometimes abbreviated as PAN.

Primary in this context simply means first. So a PAN is the first neurone or nerve in the afferent pathway. A secondary afferent neurone is the second one in the chain and so on. Sometimes the terms 'first order' or 'second order' neurone is used.

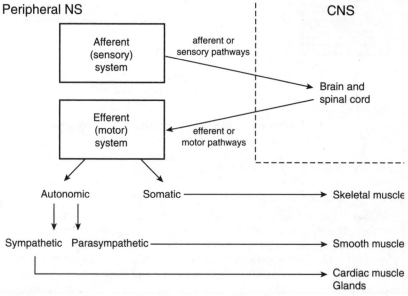

Figure 2.1 The main components of the nervous system.

The sensory part of the CNS is constantly receiving all sorts of information from the periphery and transmitting it to the CNS. It may be helpful here to review the main parts of the CNS – see Figure 2.1.

Sensory nerve fibres exist in a variety of sizes. Larger fibres conduct at a faster rate and are important for relaying information that is required urgently by the CNS – for example, where your limbs are when you are sprinting, where the pain source is that is hurting you. Smaller fibres conduct information that is not required so rapidly.

The slowest, smallest fibres are called C-fibres. They are unmyelinated, that is the fibre is not surrounded by myelin. C-fibres conduct impulses at speeds of 0.5–2.0 metres/second and conduct sensations of dull pain. The larger fibres, or A-fibres, are surrounded by a sheath of myelin, formed from concentric layers of cell membrane wound around the nerve. This myelin acts as insulation and allows greater speed of conduction; impulses are conducted at speeds of 6.0–120 meters/second. The A group is further subdivided into the α, β, γ and δ subgroups. It is the Aδ fibres that are involved in the perception of acute pain. Sharp pain is conducted rapidly by these fibres (Figure 2.2).

C-fibres may be polymodal – that is, they respond to all three types of noxious stimuli (Bogduk, 1989); but increasingly evidence suggests that a

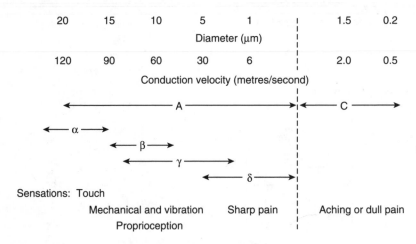

Figure 2.2　Properties of afferent nociceptive fibres.

A fibre is defined as a nociceptor when it responds to a noxious stimulus. This is a *qualitative* difference to other types of fibre, not a matter of degree. Thus, if a large Aα fibre is stimulated, it will not transmit pain. Intense stimulation of these fibres elicits a variety of descriptions of the sensation from subjects, but they do not describe 'pain'.

single fibre will preferentially respond to just one type of stimulus. C-fibres are widespread and constitute the majority of nerve fibres in many sensory nerves. The Aδ fibres are sometimes called A-mechano-heat fibres since they only respond to mechanical or thermal stimuli (Rang *et al.*, 1991). Generally speaking nociceptive fibres have a high threshold for firing – that is, they do not respond to a gentle stimulus. There is, however, a second population of low-threshold Aδ fibres that exist which respond to non-damaging pressure and can become more sensitive under certain conditions, so that small amounts of pressure can cause pain.

The other subgroups of A-fibres respond to non-nociceptive stimuli, such as touch, vibration or proprioception (where the body is in space).

Nociceptive pathways

Once a receptor has been stimulated, the information is passed along the afferent nerve to the spinal cord.

When a receptor is stimulated it causes the neurone to 'fire' – that is, the cell depolarises and an action potential of electrical energy moves along the axon effectively conveying the message from the receptor to the main part of the cell. This causes the cell to pass a message to nearby cells. Neuronal cells communicate with other neurones or muscle, endocrine cells etc. Neurones are not in direct contact; there is a small gap, or synapse, between cells. Neurotransmitters are the chemical messengers which cross this gap to facilitate the next event in the chain. A neurone may contain more than one transmitter, in which case these transmitters may be released together or separately (Figure 2.3).

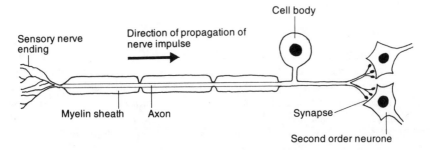

Figure 2.3 A typical sensory neurone. Information from the nerve ending travels along the myelinated axon by waves of electrical depolarisation. On reaching the nerve terminal messages are transmitted across the synapse by chemical neuro-transmitters which act at receptors on the neuronal membrane. The myelin sheath surrounding the axon aids conduction of nerve impulses. Sensory neurones have their cell body outside the spinal cord in the dorsal root ganglion.

Primary afferent nerves have their cell body in a structure called the dorsal root ganglion and enter the spinal cord via the dorsal horn or dorsal root (Figure 2.4). Nociceptive afferent nerves do not have any synapses outside the dorsal root ganglion. So, once the fibre has been activated, say in the big toe, this message will pass uninterrupted to the spinal cord. This fact is important when considering where to try and act in order to control the pain.

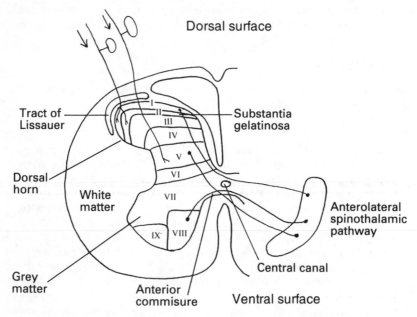

Figure 2.4 Cross-section of the spinal cord. Afferent fibres enter the cord via the dorsal horn and form synapses in different laminae of the grey matter.

After entering the spinal cord these fibres ascend or descend in a channel of tissue, called Lissauer's tract, for one or two segments before entering the grey matter and terminating in laminae I, II or V. Here they synapse with second order neurones which cross the spinal cord in the anterior commisure and ascend to the brain. So information from the right side of the body travels to the brain on the left side of the spinal cord and vice versa.

Sensory or afferent neural pathways taking information to the brain are also called ascending. Efferent or motor pathways are descending.

A cross-section of the spinal cord shows that the grey matter is organised in roughly an 'H' shape around a central canal. (The actual shape depends upon the level at which the cord is sectioned.) The grey matter is organised into layers or laminae, and it is laminae I, II and V which receive nociceptive fibres. It is beyond the scope of this book to consider the complex organisation of the spinal cord in detail. However, some important points deserve mentioning.

Lamina I (also called the marginal layer) receives inputs from Aδ mechanoreceptors and some polymodal C-fibres. The input to this region is mainly from skin and muscle nociceptors.

Lamina II (or *substantia gelatinosa*, literally meaning 'jelly substance', a reflection of the greyish jelly-like appearance of the fresh tissue) contains neurones that make local connections.

Lamina V receives inputs from Aδ-, C-fibres and non-nociceptive Aβ-fibres as well as inputs from interneurones in laminae I and II. The receptive field of lamina V is much larger than either laminae I or II. This layer is, therefore, able to convey information about pain, its location, intensity and the form of the harmful stimulus. Second order neurones which have inputs from nociceptive and non-nociceptive afferents are termed wide dynamic range (WDR) neurones. It is at this point that influences can be exerted from other parts of the body; from the periphery and from the CNS. The important parts of the CNS which influence nociceptive information include the body's own analgesic system as well as higher brain areas involved with thoughts and emotions.

This 'influencing' of nociceptive transmission is termed modulation. Modulation may involve a decrease or increase of pain perception, since both excitatory and inhibitory connections exist. This is why pain transmission is not an automatic event – it depends on the balance between excitatory and inhibitory influences on neurones in the spinal cord.

Another important point to note is that dorsal horn cells receive information from more than one afferent fibre. For example, neurones receiving inputs from deep structures (muscle, fascia, joint, tendon, bone) may also have inputs from skin or other deep tissues (Yu & Mense, 1990). These inputs will not always be from nociceptive afferents, but may be from fibres detecting non-noxious stimuli such as touch or vibration. The significance of these dual inputs to the same cell is very important in the context of referred pain and 'gating' concepts in pain perception (see below).

As the anterolateral spinothalmic tract (sometimes called the neo-spinothalamic tract) courses upwards in the spinal cord, new fibres join at each segmental level. As new fibres join, they push the fibres from more caudal levels laterally (or sideways) so that the tract is made up of layers with the longer fibres originating at the base of the spinal cord on the 'outside' and the shorter fibres from the thoracic and neck regions being more medial (or near the centre). These fibres terminate in the thalamus,

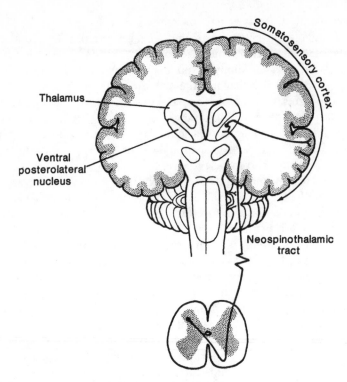

Figure 2.5   The neospinothalamic tract consists of a rapid three neurone relay system from the dorsal horn to the ventral posterolateral nucleus to the somatosensory cortex. This system allows analysis of the site, intensity and nature of the pain (see text). Reproduced from Borenstein, D.G. & Wiesel, S.W. (1989) *Low Back Pain*, pp. 25, with kind permission of W.B. Saunders Company.

particularly the ventral posterolateral nucleus, where because of the organisation of the spinothalamic tract a relationship will exist between the location of the fibre and where it originated in the body. These fibres synapse with third-order neurones which carry information to the sensory cortex (Figure 2.5). This system, therefore, allows the sensory cortex to detect pain and to analyse the site, intensity and nature of the pain. Information is also relayed to cells that provide information to the descending systems (see below).

A second ascending pathway in the spinal cord is the paleospinothalamic tract (Latin, *neo* = new; *paleo* = old – names which reflect how these tracts have developed in evolutionary terms). This tract relays information to the brainstem, the thalamus, limbic forebrain and frontal cortical structures (Figure 2.6). These are the parts of the brain involved with feelings and emotions. This pathway allows the frontal cortical responses to pain – feelings of suffering, fear, depression, anxiety, etc. These emotions are known as the 'affect' of pain.

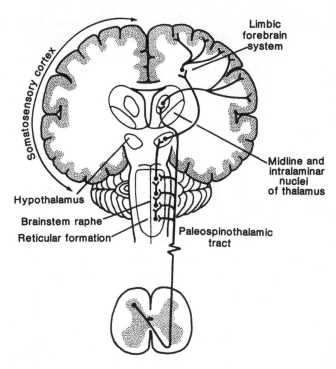

Figure 2.6 The paleospinothalamic tract consists of a slow multi-neurone relay system from the dorsal horn to the brainstem, hypothalamus and limbic forebrain. This system mediates reflexes and integrated responses (fear, memory, suffering) related to nociceptive impulses. Reproduced from Borenstein, D.G. & Wiesel, S.W. (1989) *Low Back Pain*, pp. 26, with kind permission of W.B. Saunders Company.

This pathway also has connections with neurones in the brainstem reticular formation, the hypothalamus and temporal lobe. These brain areas are involved with the descending pathways of pain control, autonomic sympathetic and parasympathetic reflexes and recent and short-term memory respectively. Thus, further opportunities are provided for complex interactions between pain and other emotions or responses to occur. Although these responses can interact, it is not obligatory that they do so. Consequently, pain does not always result in autonomic reflexes or emotions being triggered.

Pathological pain and sensitisation

Pathological pain, as we said, is characterised by a disruption of normal sensory mechanisms so that pain can occur in the absence of a clear stimulus, maybe in an exaggerated fashion or in response to normally non-noxious stimuli (Woolf, 1991). These phenomena represent an increase in sensitivity, or sensitisation. Sensitisation is an important property of nociceptors that helps us understand why innocuous stimuli become painful when disease or injury has occurred. Nociceptors may become sensitised after injury, especially after thermal injury to the skin.

Sensitisation can result in receptors becoming more sensitive with repeated application of the noxious stimulus. When this occurs each successive application of the stimulus causes the receptor to give a greater response.

When sensitisation occurs, any or all of the following can occur:

- decreased threshold of the nociceptor to activation;
- increased receptive field of nociceptors;
- response of nociceptors to normally non-noxious stimuli (allodynia);
- increased intensity of response (hyperalgesia);
- prolonged post-stimulus sensations (hyperpathia);
- emergence of spontaneous activity.

The prolongation of pain after an acute injury may actually be useful, since it causes the injured person to guard or rest the affected part of the body. Sensitisation may also help to explain the changes that occur during disease, why movement of a normal joint does not produce much sensation but movement of a joint inflamed by arthritis is painful. Sensitation also helps explain why normally we are not aware of internal organs like ovaries, the pancreas or kidneys, but if these organs are diseased or infected, then we become aware of painful sensations – although we may not always be able to localise the pain. Sadly, some-times the useful component of pain is missing – for example, one of the most insidious of diseases, cancer, usually does not cause pain in organs such as the ovaries or pancreas until it is too late for successful medical intervention. In some cases the condition may send a 'warning signal' of pain, but it is not heeded by the individual or by the clinician and its purpose is lost.

There are two components to sensitisation: peripheral and central.

Peripheral sensitisation

Tissue damage results in inflammation. Damaged cells leak cellular contents, and inflammatory cells including mast cells, macrophages, lymphocytes and polymorphonuclear leucocytes are attracted to the area of damage where they release inflammatory mediators. This 'sensitising soup' contains neuropeptides, histamine, serotonin, potassium ions, bradykinin and arachidonic acid metabolites. These agents, in turn act to alter the transduction properties of high-threshold receptors (Rang *et al.*, 1991). Low intensity stimuli, which would not normally activate noci-ceptors, now begin to do so – hence the sensitisation response. Any disease process which causes inflammation will have the potential of sensitising nociceptors and thus increasing pain. This is peripheral sensitisation. We shall see later how drugs which can act on inflammatory mediators can help in the treatment of pain (see Chapter 7).

An important observation in relation to sensitisation is that under normal circumstances a substantial number of afferents (10–40%) are 'silent' – that is, they do not normally respond to any stimuli (Woolf, 1991). Following inflammation, however, these afferents are recruited and become sensitive. Slow recruitment of a number of fibres may explain why some clinical pain builds up slowly and greatly outlasts the precipitating cause (McMahon & Koltzenburg, 1990).

Central sensitisation

A second component of sensitisation is that of central sensitisation. What essentially happens in these circumstances is that the central processing of information from the peripheral afferent nerves is altered so that fibres, especially the Aβ afferents, which are not normally nociceptors, now send messages which are interpreted as pain. Under normal circumstances the activation of low threshold Aβ afferents is by tactile stimuli, pressure to deep tissue, movements of joints, etc. which do not produce pain. After central sensitisation has occurred these sensations now cause pain. What has happened is that the cells of the dorsal horn are actually modified by the sensitising inputs and pain messages are initiated by Aβ inputs. (Woolf, 1991).

A possible site for such sensitisation are the WDR neurones, since these neurones receive both high threshold nociceptive (Aδ) and low threshold non-nociceptive (Aβ) inputs. Alterations in sensitivity of such a WDR neurone could cause the neurone to respond to Aβ fibres as if they were nociceptive fibres, and pain would be perceived in response to light touch, or other non-noxious stimuli. This would also increase the peripheral receptive field.

Central sensitisation is believed to be mediated by excitatory amino acids (e.g. glutamate and aspartate) acting at the N-methyl-D-aspartate (NMDA) receptor (Codere & Melzack,1992). Antagonists of the NMDA receptor, such as ketamine, may therefore have a role in treating such pain.

Plasticity in the CNS

An important concept in understanding how such changes can occur is the concept of plasticity in the CNS. The CNS can be described accurately in anatomical terms, but we must not assume because of this that it is an unchanging entity. Nerve cells have an inherent plasticity which means that they can modify function in response to different circumstances. This property is not restricted to nociceptive pathways – it is a property of many neurones.

Removing a normal input or severing the nerve can cause changes in neurones. For example, cells that formerly responded only to stimulation of a region of the foot may, after removal of the normal afferent input, begin to respond to stimuli applied to an area of the leg adjacent to the foot.

When peripheral nerves are damaged by injury or during surgery, they will try to grow and reinervate the area of tissue that was denervated by the destruction of the nerve. (There is no evidence for regrowth of neurones or nerves in the CNS.) These properties also contribute to the plasticity of the system. These changes are summarised in Figure 2.7.

'Wind-up'

An important concept in neuronal plasticity is that of 'wind-up'. If a recording is made of the activity of a neurone from the spinal cord, it will be seen to give a spike of activity in response to stimulus – the action potential. If, however, a series of stimuli are applied in reasonably rapid succession, the response from the neurone will be seen to increase markedly. Thus the response to the last stimulus will be greater than the response to the first stimulus even though the size of stimulus has not changed. This has important clinical implications, for if a painful stimulus is present for a long time, it will become increasingly more painful and may cause changes in the nociceptive pathway that lead to a state of hyperalgesia.

The clinical consequences of sensitisation are considered in Chapter 3.

Primary and secondary hyperalgesia

As described above, an increased sensitivity to pain or hyperalgesia occurs when nociceptive afferents have been sensitised. This primary hyperalgesia can be accompanied in some cases by a so-called secondary hyperalgesia, defined as a lowered pain threshold in the area beyond the site of injury (that is in apparently uninjured tissue). Secondary hyperalgesia is thought to result from adaptive changes in the CNS in the way that central sensitisation occurs.

The phenomena of central sensitisation has important clinical considerations since if activation of the pathway by the initial pain producing stimulus in the periphery can be avoided, then sensitisation will not occur. Although such prevention is often not possible, there are a large number of clinical situations where pain can be predicted and avoided (e.g. in surgery, before giving injections). The use of such preventative analgesia will be discussed in Chapter 7.

A second important point to remember is that if central sensitisation has occurred, any treatment which aims just to prevent nociceptor activation is bound to be inadequate (Woolf, 1991).

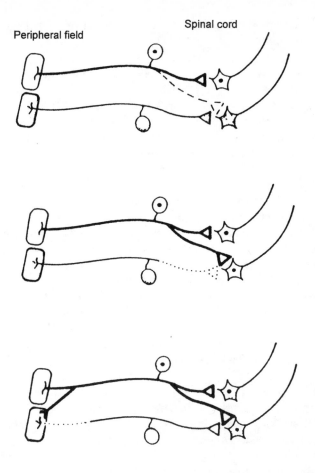

Figure 2.7 Functional plasticity of primary afferent nociceptors. **Top:** normal connectivity of primary afferents. Primary afferents innervate a defined peripheral region and activate a specific set of spinal cord neurones. Primary afferents also have central connections that are normally inactive (dashed lines). **Middle:** when the *central* process of a primary afferent that innervates an adjacent field is interrupted (dotted line) the formerly ineffective central connection of the intact primary afferent (heavy line) becomes effective. Both spinal cord cells now respond only to stimulation of innervated peripheral field. **Lower:** when the peripheral process of the adjacent primary afferent is cut (dotted line) changes occur in the spinal cord that are similar to those produced by cutting the central process. In addition the primary afferent (heavy line) sprouts and grows into the denervated peripheral region. So both spinal cord cells respond to stimulation of both peripheral fields. Reproduced from Fields, H.L. (1987) *Pain*, with kind permission of McGraw Hill Companies.

2.2 Modulation of nociceptive information – endogenous pain suppression

We have seen how information is relayed from nociceptive receptors via ascending pathways to interpretative areas in the brain (Figures 2.4 and 2.5). Information is also relayed back from the brain to the spinal cord in a descending pathway. As nociceptive afferents enter the spinal cord in the dorsal horn, they form synapses with other nerve endings. Some of these nerve endings are from neurones whose cell bodies are in the brain and whose axons form a descending pathway. These descending pathways function to modulate activity in the nociceptive pathway (Fields, 1987).

One pathway begins in the periventricular nucleus and descends via the periaqueductal grey of the midbrain to the nucleus raphe magnus in the medulla (Figure 2.8). From the nucleus raphe magnus there is a projection to the dorsal horn of the spinal cord via the dorsal longitudinal fasiculus or descending tract. This pathway terminates in the spinal cord, in laminae I, II and V to modulate nociceptive inputs. A second, more lateral, pathway originates in the nucleus reticularis gigantocellularis and a third arises in the locus coeruleus (Figure 2.8). Just how effective these pathways can be has been demonstrated by the observations of neurosurgeons who have placed electrodes in the relevant midbrain sites in humans and used electrical stimulation to produce a selective reduction of severe clinical pain (Hosobuchi *et al.*, 1977).

When the potent analgesic morphine is injected into these brain stem sites, it produces analgesia in the absence of motor, sensory or autonomic blockade, showing that a major action of morphine is to activate descending inhibitory neurones in the brainstem.

Descending pathways act by stimulating interneurones which in turn inhibit the nociceptive afferent and thus prevent the transmission of information in the nociceptive pathway.

2.3 Processing of information in the dorsal horn and the concept of 'gating' in pain pathways

The perception of pain is more than a simple equation: the greater the stimulus, the greater the pain. Pain perception is a complex and subtle process. In dramatic situations quite severe wounds can go unnoticed, or in other circumstances prolonged and persistent pain can sometimes not be traced to any organic cause. Destruction of peripheral nerves – which might be thought to totally remove a component of the nociceptive pathway and therefore the route of nociceptive input – often results, paradoxically, in enduring pain. Amputated limbs can give a phantom limb pain, or arms rendered inactive by brachial plexus avulsion can continue to be a source of worrying pain for the sufferer. Thus pain

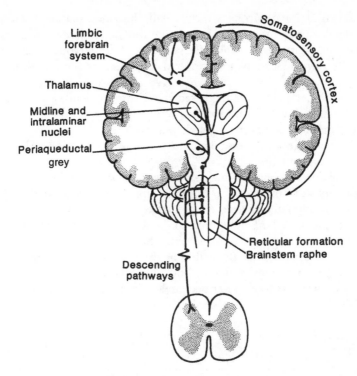

Figure 2.8 Descending pathways from the brain. These pathways carry signals from higher brain centres through the periaqueductal grey matter and the brainstem back to the dorsal horn, where they can influence nociceptive transmission. Reproduced from Borenstein, D.G. & Wiesel, S.W. (1989) *Low Back Pain*, pp. 27, with kind permission of W.B. Saunders Company.

perception is more complex than the stimulation of the pathway and the production of a result. Just why pain alters under different circumstances and with different individuals is one of the great mysteries in the understanding of pain.

One of the original and most famous attempts to explain why pain perception is so complex was Melzack and Wall's development of the 'Gate Control Theory' in 1965. Even though the concept of a 'gating event' is useful in understanding how pain can be so variable, the theory can now be seen to be incomplete and even incorrect in some detail (Fields, 1987). What is meant by gating is that transmission of a nociceptive stimulus is not an 'all-or-nothing' event; it may be modified by other events in the nervous system.

Nociceptive information is relayed from the periphery to the spinal cord by small diameter Aδ and C-fibres, which synapse with second order neurones and also interneurones in the dorsal horn of the spinal cord. These dorsal horn cells also receive non-noxious input from other fibres. It is probably these interneurones which provide the conceptual site of the 'gate' (although many scientists would argue that we cannot identify uneqivocally just which cells are responsible – the plasticity of the nervous system means that cells may change how they respond depending on the circumstances).

For example, if a dorsal horn cell receives input from a nociceptive and a non-nociceptive fibre, then increased activity in the non-nociceptive fibre may 'dampen down' the nociceptive activity. So if we rub a painful spot, the rubbing signals may get through and block the pain signals. This may be why massage and transcutaneous electrical stimulation (TENS) are useful to control pain.

A large non-myelinated fibre could have a constant inhibitory influence on nociceptive transmission. If this large fibre is damaged, there will be a loss of inhibition and therefore a greater experience of pain.

There could be both inhibitory and excitatory interneurones, so the possibilities of different messages being relayed are endless.

It is not clear whether the action at the interneurones is presynaptic, postsynaptic or a combination of both. Actions at presynaptic terminals would result in less transmitter being released. Postsynaptic actions might involve altering the level of excitability of interneurones to arriving nerve impulses, making them either hyperpolarised and easily excited or hypo-polarised and less sensitive to nerve impulses.

A presynaptic terminal is *before* the synapse, so activity here would influence how much transmitter is released to cross the synapse. Postsynaptic refers to the membrane *after* the synapse – that is, the one receiving messages from the neurotransmitter. Changes here would affect how a cell responds to the same message, either by increased or decreased activity.

This gives us a conceptual framework to understand why pain trans-mission is so variable. Imagine a situation where the sensitivity of the interneurone is changed. The whole nociceptive pathway could be extre-mely sensitive, giving rise to phenomena such as allodynia (permanent, inappropriate pain). Under other circumstances the whole system could be inhibited, resulting in an insensitivity to pain. Rather than a 'gate' that it only open or closed, it might be easier to envisage the spinal cord as the volume knob on a radio: it could be turned down very low so that the sound was almost inaudible or turned up so loud that the sound would be unbearably deafening.

Using this analogy we might envisage pain management as trying to turn the radio off. If, however, this is not possible then perhaps turning the volume down as low as possible and also making a louder noise or some other distraction, elsewhere, will also make the radio inaudible.

Thus a combination of analgesic drugs, surgical techniques and non-invasive measures may succeed where a single intervention alone is not enough.

2.4 Transmitters in nociceptive pathways

If we are to have some influence over the pain pathway and employ intelligent use of analgesic drugs, an understanding of which neurotransmitters can be identified in the nociceptive pathway is crucial, as is an examination of how they can be modified by pharmacological intervention. Because such a complex area of neuropharmacology cannot be covered in any detail in this work, this section highlights the main transmitters and concentrates on those which help our understanding of analgesic drugs.

Histochemical analysis of the dorsal horn region and the dorsal root ganglion (DRG) reveal that there are a very large number of peptides and excitatory amino acids present. Some have been clearly identified as nociceptive transmitters, some may act as facilitatory transmitters and others have a status of 'possible' transmitters (Yaksh & Malmberg, 1994). The situation is even more complex, as many neurones contain more than one transmitter and the neurotransmitters of importance may vary with the peripheral site innervated. This means that activation of a primary afferent may send a more complex signal. For example, a fast acting excitatory amino acid may be released along with a peptide which could have a more enduring postsynaptic activity. So an immediate signal, causing a rapid response from the nociceptive pathway, may be followed by a more prolonged, less intense signal.

The most predominant transmitter in the nociceptive pathway is substance P, an 11 amino acid peptide. Histochemistry has shown that approximately 80% of the DRG cells contain substance P, around 50% of cells containing both substance P and CGRP (calcitonin gene related peptide) (Ju *et al.*, 1987). Also important is the excitatory amino acid glutamate. Other important neurotransmitters are the excitatory amino acid aspartate and peptides such as VIP (vasoactive intestinal polypeptide), somatostatin, CCK (cholecystokinin), and endorphins.

More is known about the transmitters of the descending pathways where the main transmitters are serotonin, noradrenaline and opiates, although other peptides are also found (Yaksh & Malmberg, 1994).

Descending tracts from the periaqueductal grey and raphe are thought to release serotonin which activates interneurones in lamina V of the spinal cord. The interneurone inhibits the nociceptors that produce substance P. Thus active transmission of the nociceptive information is effectively blocked. The transmitter used by these interneurones is enkephalin, one of the family of opiates (Figure 2.9).

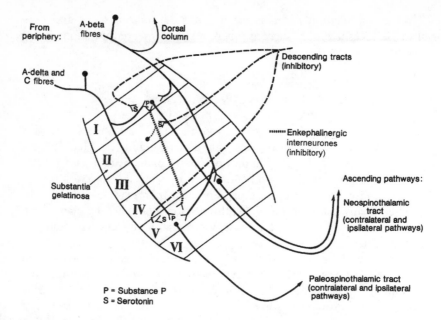

Figure 2.9 Organisation of the pain-related fibres in the dorsal horn. Nociceptive Aδ and C-fibres carry messages from the periphery to laminae I and V. These neurones synapse with second order relay neurones, which ascend in the neospinothalamic or paleospinothalamic tracts. Nociceptive messages in these neurones are modified presynaptically by collateral branches of large low-threshold fibres (Aβ). Nociceptive fibres are also inhibited by enkephalins or serotonin. See text for more detail. Reproduced from Borenstein, D.G. & Wiesel, S.W. (1989) *Low Back Pain*, pp. 24, with kind permission of W.B. Saunders Company.

Descending pathway inhibition can be shown to rely on opiate receptors for its action since naloxone, an opiate antagonist, temporarily reverses the analgesic effect of activation of the periaqueductal grey or raphe neurones.

The importance of serotonin is that it produces analgesia when applied directly to the spinal cord, and the destruction of the serotoninergic neurones is accompanied by a reduction in the analgesic action of brainstem stimulation.

Although the nor-adrenergic pathways have not been as clearly defined as the serotoninergic pathways, there are a large number of neurones in the lateral and dorsal pons which project to the spinal cord containing noradrenaline, and it is likely that some of these project to the dorsal horn. Direct intrathecal application of agonists of noradrenaline, in primates, has been found to block responses to noxious stimuli (Duggan, 1985).

Drugs that affect the pharmacological actions of serotonin and noradrenaline can have analgesic activity. Tricyclic antidepressants, such as amitriptyline, block the presynaptic uptake of both serotonin and noradrenaline, thus augmenting their postsynaptic action in descending pathways, although it is not universally accepted that this is how they act as analgesics. It is interesting to note that antidepressant activity may take days or weeks to be noticeable, whereas analgesic activity can be quite rapid.

WITHDRAWN

Neurotransmitters act on receptors to produce their action. This action is terminated when the transmitter is destroyed or when it diffuses away from the receptor and is taken up by the nerve ending from which it was originally released. This process is called re-uptake. If a re-uptake inhibitor is present, this mechanism is inhibited and the neurotransmitter remains in the synaptic space. It will continue to interact with receptors and thereby prolong its action.

2.5 Descending pathways and endogenous opiates

Although serotonin, noradrenaline and opiates are all important in the descending pathways that modulate pain perception, it is worth considering the opiates in more detail since so many of the pharmacological interventions used to treat pain rely on the use of opioid analgesics, which mimic the action of endogenous opiates.

Naturally occurring derivatives of morphine found in the opium poppy are termed opiates. Synthetic, semi-synthetic and natural compounds are encompassed in the broader term opioids.

Perhaps our oldest and most potent analgesic drug is morphine, one of the components of the sap of the opium poppy *Papaver somniferum*, known collectively as opiates. Originally discovered by the Chinese, the analgesic and euphoric properties of opium have been known for over 2000 years.

Opiates were shown to produce analgesia by acting on opioid receptors (these are covered in detail in Chapter 7, when opioid drugs are discussed). The discovery of opiate receptors was so important because the presence of these receptors in the body meant that there must be substances in the body that will combine with these receptors – in other words the body must produce its own natural opiates.

Most biologically active messenger substances, like hormones, neurotransmitters and so on, produce their action by combining with receptors. An easy way to envisage a biological messenger and its receptor is to think of a lock and key. The active messenger is the key, its precise size and shape determines which lock – or receptor – it will fit into. A key can only open its own lock and, similarly, a transmitter will only activate its own receptor. Once activated a receptor produces a biological response – that is, the cell is prompted to do something: a neurone would fire, a muscle cell contract, etc. In receptor terminology the key is called a ligand. A ligand that produces a normal biological response is an agonist; whereas a ligand that prevents a normal response is an antagonist (the key sits in the lock, but it won't turn).

These naturally occurring analgesics were proposed by Terenius and colleagues (Terenius *et al.*, 1973), isolated in 1975 (Hughes *et al.*, 1975) and termed endorphins (endogenous morphine) and enkephalins (endogenous opiates in the kephalus – Greek for brain).

There are three major groups of endogenous opiates:

- the enkephalins – leucine-enkephalin (leu-enkephalin) and methionine-enkephalin (met-enkephalin);
- β-endorphin;
- the dynorphins – dynorphin and α-neoendorphin.

The enkephalins and endorphins are derived from a larger precursor molecule (Figure 2.10). Endorphin is made by enzymatic cleavage of pro-opiomelanocortin (POMC), a molecule which produces adrenocorticotrophic hormone (ACTH), melanocyte stimulating hormone (α-MSH) and lipotrophins. Proenkephalin gives several copies of met-enkephalin and leu-enkephalin. Pro-dynorphin produces α-neo endorphin and dynorphin.

Opiates produce analgesia by a direct action on the CNS. Injection of small amounts of opiates directly into the brain can produce potent analgesia. Animal experiments mapping the most sensitive sites of opiate analgesia have shown that the periaqueductal grey and the medulla are highly sensitive to morphine (see Reisine & Pasternak, 1996).

Analgesia can be induced by electrical stimulation, and the brainstem regions which are most sensitive correspond largely to those which respond to opiate microinjection. This has led to the proposal that systemically administered opiates, such as morphine, produce analgesia by activation of the descending nociceptive modulating system. Opiate antagonists, such as naloxone, when injected into these regions (periaqueductal grey or rostroventral medulla) can antagonise the analgesic action of systemic opiates (Fields, 1987).

Enkephalin, as described above, is important in interneurones which

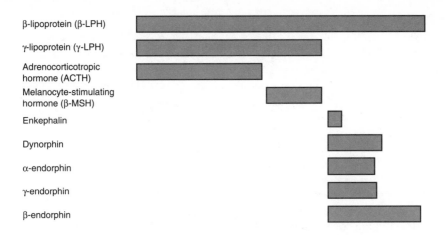

β-lipoprotein (β-LPH)

γ-lipoprotein (γ-LPH)

Adrenocorticotropic hormone (ACTH)

Melanocyte-stimulating hormone (β-MSH)

Enkephalin

Dynorphin

α-endorphin

γ-endorphin

β-endorphin

Figure 2.10 The pro-opiomelanocortin family of peptides. The parent molecule, β-lipotropin, is cleaved enzymically to give rise to the adrenocorticotrophic hormone (ACTH) family of peptides and the endorphin and enkephalin family of peptides.

inhibit substance P release and thus stops transmission of nociceptive information.

Potentiation has been observed between opioids and adrenergic agonists, although no such potentiation has been seen with serotonin.

This may have implications for the co-administration of antidepressants and opioids, since anti-depressants such as amitriptyline act by increasing the noradrenaline available and thus may lower the level of morphine required.

Potentiation occurs when the effect of two drugs given together is greater than what would be achieved from the effect of each one. One drug potentiates the activity of the other.

The endorphins and enkephalins are found in all the brain and spinal cord structures involved in nociception, although there are differences in the anatomical distribution of each family of endogenous opiates.

These effects of morphine have been demonstrated in animals and in humans by using experimentally induced pain. However, it has often been noted that in the clinical situation morphine seems to have effects that are more complex and subtle than can be explained by these pathways alone – that is, morphine can alter the sensation of pain and the affective response to the pain. Patients report that the pain is still present, but they feel more comfortable (Reisine & Pasternak, 1996).

2.6 Opiates and gene expression

The naturally occurring opiates exist to provide the body with a means of suppressing pain. It has been shown that one response to inflammation is to increase the production of endogenous opiates. This has been shown under experimental conditions where inflammation at peripheral sites causes a marked increase in preprodynorphin messenger riboxynucleic acid (mRNA) and preproenkephalin mRNA (Iadorola *et al.*, 1988). Thus production of leu-enkephalin, met-enkephalin and dynorphin are increased (Draisci & Iadorola, 1989).

Messenger RNA is the biochemical intermediate between DNA and the peptide or protein made under the control of that DNA. DNA determines the sequence of mRNA which thus determines the sequence of amino acids that are assembled to form a peptide or protein. In this case the peptide is preprodynorphin which is cleaved to give dynorphin or preproenkephalin which is cleaved to enkephalin (see Figure 2.10).

This increase in the natural opiates occurs in neurones in laminae I–II and V–VI of the spinal cord, where, as discussed, enkephalins can inhibit substance P and thus decrease transmission in the nociceptive pathway. Furthermore, exogeneously administered opioids are known to influence the regulation and expression of opioid genes (Crosby *et al.*, 1994). This raises the possibility that pharmacological manipulation of gene expression might provide a novel method of pain control.

Summary of Chapter 2

- Pain varies under different circumstances.
- Pain may be viewed as either physiological or pathological.
- Perception of pain involves four processes:

  - transduction
  - transmission
  - modulation
  - perception
- Nociceptive information is received by chemical, mechanical or thermal receptors.
- Different nerve fibres are involved in the transmission of nociceptive information.
- C-fibres are slow conducting and transmit dull pain.
- Aδ-fibres are faster conducting and transmit sharp pain.
- Nociceptive information is transmitted from the periphery to the spinal cord and then to the brain.
- It is only when nociceptive information is interpreted by the brain that the sensation of pain is felt.
- There are many points along the transmission pathway where information may be modified.
- Pathological pain is characterised by a disruption of normal sensory mechanisms so the pain occurs in the absence of a clear stimulus.
- This increased sensitivity means that normally innocuous stimuli now cause pain.
- Increased sensitivity can occur in the periphery or centrally.
- The body possesses endogenous analgesics – endorphins, enkephalins and dynorphins which can be 'turned on' to control pain.

Chapter 3

The Causes of Clinical Pain

It is clearly impossible to cover all the potential sources of pain that can be encountered in a nursing context. Understanding the physiology of pain, however, gives a broad framework for gaining some insight into how many diseases cause pain. Any inflammation will release chemical inflammatory modulators which can act directly on nociceptors to produce pain. Tissue swelling due to oedema, a disease process or a tumour will produce mechanical distortion and pain. Nerves can be damaged, compressed, pinched, trapped or infiltrated by diseased tissue (especially cancer metastases), and these can all cause pain. We have also seen how these primary nociceptive events can in turn lead to changes in the CNS which make formerly innocuous stimuli produce pain and how a long-term painful state can be induced. (You may need to refer to Chapter 2 when reading the following sections.)

This chapter deals first with specific types of pain that may occur in many different diseases and then outlines some of the more commonly encountered painful conditions – cancer pain, post-operative pain, post-herpetic neuralgia, angina, trigeminal neuralgia, migraine, arthritis, labour pain, burn pain, pelvic and back pain. There are also sections on treatment-related pain and miscellaneous pains experienced by bedridden patients. This list is certainly not exhaustive and there are some areas of pain that are not covered; but information on pain and the pain literature are too vast to be covered in a book of this size. The approach has been to include the most common painful conditions, and concentrate on those where analgesic medication features prominently in treatment.

Part 1. Specific types of pain

This section outlines some of the important features of the more common types of pathological pain. There is always a problem in trying to categorise a particular pain, for many different terminologies are used in the literature. No single universal system for classifying pain exists; remember too that a single pain may fall into more than one category or may be described by several different terms. Table 3.1 at the end of this section summarises the salient features of the different terms used here. The types of pain included are:

- neuropathic pain (this includes sympathetically maintained pain, reflex sympathetic dystrophy, deafferentation, central pain, peripheral neuropathy);
- somatic, cutaneous, and visceral;
- acute pain and chronic pain;
- chronic pain syndrome;
- referred pain;
- radicular pain;
- phantom limb and stump pain;
- breakthrough pain;
- intractable pain.

3.1 Neuropathic pain

Neuropathic (also called neurogenic or deafferentation) pain does not require the presence of an identifiable noxious stimulus. In several articles or books pain is considered in two categories – as nociceptive and neuropathic pain, with nociceptive defined as pain in response to an obvious stimulus, while neuropathic is defined as pain in the absence of such a stimulus. (Nociceptive pain was described in Chapter 2.) Neuropathic pain may be baffling to patient and healthcare professionals alike, as there is no obvious noxious stimulus present. It can be long-lasting and unpleasant and is variously described as burning, dull, aching, boring. Episodes of sharp shooting pain, termed lancinating pain, are also experienced. Neuropathic pain results from current or past damage to the peripheral and/or central nervous system, and is due to aberrant processing of information in the peripheral or central nervous system. Neuropathic pain can be described in terms of the characteristics of the pain, the site of injury, or the presumed site of aberrant neural activity that is producing the pain.

Central mechanisms are believed to underlie two important syndromes: sympathetically maintained pain and deafferentation pain. Peripheral neuropathic pain is caused by injury to a peripheral nerve and this is the mechanism believed to be involved in those pains termed 'peripheral neuropathies'. Other factors which can cause neuropathic pain are spontaneous activity in neurones which have lost normal nociceptive input – for example, after brachial plexus avulsion.

Damaging or trapping a nerve will obviously cause an immediate, acute pain. After damage has occurred there are several ways in which damage results in continuing pain. Damaged nerves are apt to fire spontaneously, giving sudden bursts of pain. If peripheral nerves are cut or damaged, they start to regenerate by sprouting. In this way the body could be re-innervating the region that was denervated by the tissue damage. Chapter 2 discusses how such regeneration can lead to changes in the nociceptive pathways that contribute to pathological pain. It is a common experience after tissue damage, such as a deep cut, that the healing process is accompanied by a period of hyperalgesia (increased sensitivity to pain). This hyperalgesia is due to the proliferation of regenerating (regrowing) nerve fibres. In some cases these sprouting nerves cannot successfully re-innervate the tissue, and a tangle of nerve fibres is formed, called a neuroma (*pl.* neuromata). If a neuroma forms on a nociceptive axon, it can be a constant source of pain. Neuromata may be spontaneously active, giving an unexpected burst of pain, but are also at times highly sensitive to mechanical stimuli and to circulating agents, especially noradrenaline. Clinically, neuromata can give rise to stump pain, phantom limb pain, local wound pain after surgery and the central pain syndrome.

Damaged nerve endings also have altered physiological properties compared with normal afferents and become very sensitive to direct mechanical stimulation. Light tapping of the growing tip of a regenerating nerve will produce a tingling sensation (Tinel's sign). Movements that stretch or compress such a nerve can produce sudden shooting, lancinating pains. Regenerating neurones also show spontaneous activity, and pain will be felt with no apparent cause. Spontaneous activity can also occur near to the cell body in the DRG (Figure 3.1).

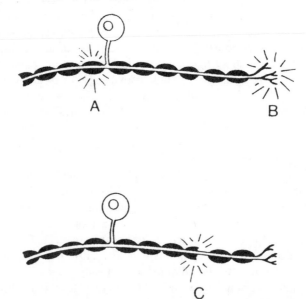

Figure 3.1 Sites of ectopic discharge in damaged primary afferent nociceptors. **Top:** a transected nerve begins to regenerate, sending out sprouts that are mechanically sensitive, sensitive to α-adrenergic agonists, and spontaneously active. In addition, a secondary site of hyperactivity (A) develops near the cell body in the DRG. **Bottom:** ectopic impulses may arise from a short patch of demyelination on a primary afferent (C). Reproduced from Fields, H.L. (1987) *Pain*, with kind permission of McGraw Hill Companies.

Damage to the myelin sheath that does not sever the nerve itself can be sufficient to cause ectopic discharge and neuropathic pain (Fields, 1987). When such damage is present the pain may be intensified, for a single impulse arriving at the demyelinated patch may produce multiple discharges in the nerve with a resultant 'stab' of pain. This mechanism has been proposed as the underlying pathology in trigeminal neuralgia (tic douloureux). Entrapment of nerves can also cause neuropathic pain.

Neuropathic pain may be more difficult to treat with analgesics than nociceptive pain. It is often opioid insensitive (Arner & Meyerson, 1988; Portenoy *et al.*, 1990).

The most common types of neuropathic pain are summarised in Table 3.1 and discussed in more detail below.

Table 3.1 Types of neuropathic pain.

Type of neuropathic pain	Cause	Features
Sympathetically maintained pain	Nociceptive efferents sensitive to sympathetic activity as a result of damage	Intense burning pain Muscle tenderness Glossy, mottled skin Pallor, cold limbs
RSDS	Sympathetic pain of the joints	Involves distal parts of limbs
Central pain	Damage to the CNS thalamus or spinal cord	Pain on the opposite side of the body to the lesion Burning, soreness, aching, sensation of 'sitting on rocks'
Deafferentation pain	Trauma which removes or damages nerves, e.g. brachial plexus avulsion	Constant intractable pain and loss of use of limb
Peripheral neuropathies	Death of a neurone or axon Loss of myelin sheath	Pain, muscular weakness and wasting Parasthesiae, tingling, burning
Phantom limb and stump pain	Neuromata formation changes in the CNS	Tingling is dominant. Also cramping, shooting or burning pain

Sympathetically maintained pain

The sympathetic nervous system is part of the efferent arm of the nervous system supplying the autonomic regulation of the body – that is, the functions of the body which occur without conscious effort, such as heartbeat, breathing, etc. The sympathetic nervous system would not be expected, therefore, to contribute to nociception. Indeed, in the normal individual this is the case, but in some circumstances a sympathetically maintained pain occurs, where normal efferent activity in the sympathetic nervous system causes pain.

Sympathetically maintained, or sympathetic dependent, pain is less well understood than nociceptive or neuropathic pain, and can complicate nociceptive or neuropathic pain. Although we do not totally understand sympathetically maintained pain, it is thought that nociceptive afferents become sensitive to sympathetic afferent activity as a result of damage to the nerves. After nerve damage, regenerating sprouts of the nociceptive nerve are thought to become sensitive to noradrenaline (the transmitter of the sympathetic nervous system). We do not know why or how this occurs. The fibres may also make artificial electrical junctions or *ephapses* with regenerating sympathetic nerves. Then what would normally be efferent activity in the sympathetic nervous system would also activate afferent nociceptive pathways (Figure 3.2).

Causalgia is the most dramatic form of sympathetically maintained pain and the first example of this type of pain to be described. It is characterised by an intense, burning pain sensation of a limb where nerve injury has occurred. The involvement of the sympathetic nervous system was demonstrated because sympathetic blockade (completely stopping transmission in the sympathetic nerve by, for example, freezing) could be shown to produce complete and immediate relief from the pain; and electrical stimulation of the sympathetic pathways could exacerbate the pain. In normal individuals sympathetic stimulation does not evoke pain, and sympathetic blockade does not impair pain sensations.

Sympathetically maintained pain is characterised by painful hypersensitivity of the skin (hyperalgesia), a sensitivity to non-noxious stimuli (allodynia), muscle tenderness, swelling of soft tissue and smooth glossy skin with a mottled appearance. Evidence of increased activity in the sympathetic nervous system is manifested as increased sweating and vasoconstriction, causing pallor and coldness of the limbs.

There is a particular type of sympathetic pain that affects joints. It is known by an extraordinary large number of different names, which probably reflects an initial lack of knowledge of the underlying cause of the condition. Thus the condition has been known as algodystrophy, Sudeck's atrophy, Sudeck's posttraumatic osteodystrophy, reflex sympathetic dystrophy syndrome (RSDS), posttraumatic sympathetic atrophy, posttraumatic painful osteoporosis, shoulder-hand syndrome or minor causalgia. In 1995 a concensus conference in the USA suggested that the umberella term 'complex regional pain syndrome (CRPS)' should be used with subdivisions into type I, corresponding to RSDS without an identifiable nerve lesion and type II, which corresponds to causalgia with an identifiable nerve lesion (Stanton-Hicks *et al.*, 1995). These terms have

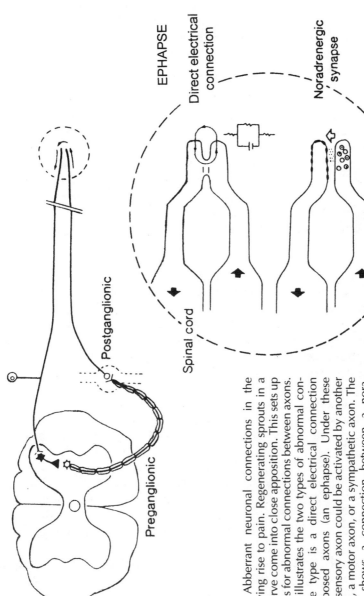

Figure 3.2 Abberrant neuronal connections in the periphery giving rise to pain. Regenerating sprouts in a peripheral nerve come into close apposition. This sets up the conditions for abnormal connections between axons. Enlargement illustrates the two types of abnormal connection. One type is a direct electrical connection between apposed axons (an ephapse). Under these conditions a sensory axon could be activated by another sensory axon, a motor axon, or a sympathetic axon. The enlargement shows a connection between a noradrenergic sympathetic postganglionic axon and a primary afferent. Reproduced from Fields, H.L. (1987) *Pain*, with kind permission of McGraw Hill Companies.

been included in the 2nd edition of the IASP classification of Chronic Pain Syndromes (see below), although any of the terms listed may be encountered.

The condition involves the distal parts of limbs, although it is well recognised to occur in the knee or shoulder and has been reported in both the hip and spine. The elbow is the least commonly involved limb joint. When the shoulder alone is involved, it is termed 'frozen shoulder', whereas when the shoulder and hand are involved, it is called shoulder–hand syndrome.

The onset is usually gradual with increasing pain in the affected joint or joints. It can occur after trauma, and the pain is usually more long lasting and severe than would be expected from the initial precipitating event. Hand–shoulder involvement can occur after myocardial infarction. The pain is variable, generally starting with pain on movement but becoming progressively more constant. In the hand pain radiates to affect the whole hand and wrist. The intensity and nature of the pain varies from a dull ache to the extreme pain of causalgia with paroxysms of lancinating pain which can be completely incapacitating (Atkins & Duthie, 1987).

Cardiovascular effects are also seen. Early in the syndrome there is a 'hot phase' where the skin is warm, red and swollen. This is followed by a 'cold phase' when the skin assumes a cool, clammy and cyanosed appearance. Finally this vasomotor instability disappears, but the skin may still retain a shiny, swollen and discoloured or mottled appearance.

Treatment is with physiotherapy to maintain passive joint movement and to encourage active use of the affected limb, although there is no evidence that physiotherapy *per se* affects the underlying pathology and natural history of the disease.

Sympathetic blockade with local anaesthetics may be useful, but success is inversely proportional to the time that elapses before treatment. Responses to this intervention also show that we do not completely understand the syndrome. The most noticeable effect is that the response to blockade outlasts the duration of action of the local anaesthetic. For example, xylocaine has a duration of action of 2 to 3 hours. It is not unusual for a patient with RSDS to have 12 hours of relief following xylocaine block. In some cases with repeated blocks the relief lasts progressively longer, finally resolving for weeks, months or even permanently.

Nonsteroidal anti-inflammatory drugs (NSAIDs) are more effective at pain relief than opioid analgesics, and benzodiazepines may be useful.

Sympathetically maintained pain occurs in cancer patients secondarily to malignant involvement of the para-aortic lymph nodes, particularly with carcinoma of the cervix or rectum. Pancreatic cancer pain and that arising from other upper abdominal viscera, such as the liver, may also have a sympathetic dependent component.

Central pain syndrome or thalamic pain

Pain due to damage in the CNS is termed central pain. The most common and debilitating example is the thalamic pain syndrome described by Dejerine and Roussy in 1906. It is thought to occur when the ventroposterolateral nucleus in the thalamus is damaged. This is the region of the brain that receives the input of the neospinothalamic tract and is, therefore, one of the cardinal components of nociceptive pathways. The cause of the damage is not always known, but a thrombosis of the inferior cerebellar artery has been identified as one of the causes.

Central pain may also be caused by pathological conditions of the spinal cord – for example, syringomyelia or tumours of the spinal cord. In this condition pain comes on gradually, sometimes over several years. The pain is on the opposite side of the body to the lesion (remember that the axons of second order neurones cross the spinal cord in the anterior commissure) and may involve the entire half of the body, only the forequarter or hindquarter or may be restricted to one limb. Where central pain involves the face, there is usually severe pain in the eye, which has been described as 'feeling as if an eye were being torn out' (Nathan, 1988). In a few cases central pain is restricted to one side of the mouth and lateral side of the hand.

With central lesions there can be any type of pain: burning, soreness, aching or a sensation of sitting or lying on rocks (Nathan, 1988). As well as constant pain any sort of stimulation can increase the pain in the affected region.

Central pains also occurs with tumours of the spinal cord, in multiple sclerosis, paraplegia and paraparesis. In multiple sclerosis the pain is aching, burning or girdle pain. In paraplegic conditions the pain is usually described as deep, boring, burning, constricting or shooting.

Deafferentation pain

When the normal nerve input is interrupted changes take place in the nervous system in response to this sensory loss. This is termed deafferentation pain (literally de = removing afferentation = the normal afferent input). It is commonly seen after brachial plexus avulsion when trauma to the arm has damaged many nerves in the complex brachial plexus of the shoulder, or it may be caused by Pancoast's tumour of the lung. The damaged arm can become useless and often quite painful. Brachial plexus avulsion is seen after instances such as motorcycle accidents and similar severe trauma.

Two processes are thought to occur in this condition. The removal of the afferent input causes an up-regulation of the normal nociceptive pathway and concomitantly the usual input from non-nociceptive fibres, which would inhibit pain responses, has been lost.

Treatment by sympathetic blockade may be helpful. Success has been reported with naloxone and physostigmine but results are variable. Clonazepam and other centrally acting drugs may be useful.

Peripheral neuropathies

Conditions which result in the death of a neurone, with the loss of the cell body and axon, are termed neuropathies. These conditions may be focal or generalised. Focal lesions occur as a result of trauma or ischaemia; generalised conditions may be due to toxins, metabolic disturbances, especially diabetes, nutritional deficiencies, such as lack of the B vitamins, or disease.

Where axonal damage has occurred but the cell body is unaffected, it is possible that axons can regenerate. Axonal regeneration is slow and itself may give rise to painful conditions, such as neuromata.

Other neuropathies primarily affect the Schwann cells and give rise to demyelination (loss of the insulating myelin sheath), without damaging the nerve axon. Such lesions are seen in multiple sclerosis or the Guillain-Barré syndrome.

Peripheral neuropathies are divided into two main categories: mononeuropathy and polyneuropathy. Mononeuropathies involve a lesion of an isolated nerve, although more than one nerve can be affected (multiple mononeuropathy). Diffuse and bilaterally symmetrical lesions give rise to polyneuropathy, where several nerves on both sides of the body are affected. Although this may sound confusing, the difference is easier to understand when the cause is considered. Polyneuropathy is most likely to be caused by metabolic disturbances, toxic agents, deficiency states and certain cases of immune reactions, which affect both sides of the body equally. By contrast, isolate nerve lesions arise from trauma, malignant conditions, nerve entrapment, thermal or electrical injury, radiation damage or vascular causes, which can be quite localised.

Neuropathies present with a variety of symptoms that will depend on which nerves have been affected. Loss of motor nerve function will cause muscular weakness and wasting. Loss of tendon reflexes is a common accompaniment to peripheral neuropathy.

Sensory nerve loss can result in decreased sensation of pain and temperature, and a consequent increase in the amount of damage sustained by the individual. Persistent ulceration, accidental damage, tissue loss – particularly in the feet – and neuropathic joint degeneration can all occur.

Parasthesiae are a frequent feature of peripheral neuropathy. They may be tingling (pins and needles), or may have a more burning quality and are aggravated by touching or rubbing the skin. Excessive or hyperpathic responses develop and normally innocent stimuli cause pain. Repeated stimulation at the same site may cause the pain to reach intolerable levels. A symptom sometimes encountered is 'restless legs' (Ekbom's syndrome) where patients experience unpleasant sensations in the legs. They are usually unable to describe the sensations precisely and may not describe pain, but find that moving their legs brings relief and hence a constant pattern of leg movement is seen.

Phantom limb and stump pain

Amputation of a limb is almost invariably followed by the feeling that the amputated part of the limb is still present, a phenomenon termed phantom limb, which may be painful. Where pain occurs at the site of scarring after amputation, it is referred to as stump pain. Stump pain is often due to neuromata formation at the site of the nerve section. While phantom limb phenomena are almost universal consequences of amputation, there is no consensus on the incidence of pain with phantom limb sensations – reports varying from 0 to 100%! (Jensen *et al.*, 1983). The underlying mechanisms are not clear but have been ascribed to a peripheral origin in the severed nerves (Sunderland, 1978), to changes in the spinal cord (Carlen *et al.*, 1978) or in the brain (Melzack, 1992). The use of epidural anaesthesia before surgery may reduce the incidence of subsequent stump pain. The mechanisms of this action are discusssed in section 3.12.

When there is a recurrence of pain in an amputated limb after surgical removal for cancer, it could signal recurrence of the tumour and must be investigated thoroughly (Foley, 1993).

3.2 Somatic, cutaneous and visceral pain

Pain sensitive structures can be divided into three main areas: the skin, the musculoskeletal system and the internal organs. Pain in the musculo-skeletal system is called somatic, and sometimes the term 'superficial somatic' is used for pain in the skin.

> The body can be divided into the soma (Greek for body) and the viscera. The soma comprises bones, periosteum, tendons and fascia, while the viscera comprises the internal organs.

The pain arising from skin is usually quite different in nature from that arising from deeper tissues. Pain sensations evoked in skin are sharp and well localised. The skin is richly supplied with both Aδ and C-fibres, and skin responds to all types of noxious stimuli. Much clinical research into pain uses cutaneous pain since the skin is so accessible, but it is usually pain from deeper tissues that presents the most pressing clinical problems. Pain in the skin can be referred pain (see below).

Muscle is less densely innervated than skin and nociceptive inputs from muscle are subject to stronger descending inhibition than is the input from cutaneous nociceptors (Yu & Mense, 1990), so muscle pain is likely to be less intense and less sharp than skin pain. Most musculoskeletal pain (or myofascial pain) is difficult to localise with the exception of pain from fascia or periosteum which is often located in a single spot (Staff, 1988). Free nerve endings in muscle are typically associated with the walls of arterioles and the surrounding connective tissue; capillaries are not supplied with nociceptive nerve endings and so are insensitive to pain (Stacey, 1969). Blood-borne agents or disturbances in the circulation will have immediate effects on nociceptive fibres. For example, lactate accumulation during anaerobic exercise will produce pain in skeletal muscle (the 'burn' of certain types of work-outs) and peripheral vascular disease can cause pain.

Ischaemia is a potent stimulus in muscle fibres and contributes to the pain of cardiac ischaemia.

Another source of myofascial pain is muscle spasm. If one muscle group is under constant tension – perhaps due to anxiety or as a consequence of pain in another part of the body, or pain in the muscle itself – it may eventually cause that muscle to go into spasm producing pain. The pain radiates in a typical distribution for each muscle group and can sometimes be felt as a tight band which is exquisitely tender. Pressure on a particular area can reproduce the pain and is called a trigger point. For a detailed discussion of trigger points, see Travel and Simmons (1983).

Cartilage is completely free of nociceptors, and pain does not arise from cartilaginous tissue directly. The periosteum or membrane surrounding bone is rich in nerve endings and any damage, stretching or distortion of the periosteum is very painful. This can happen after fractures, in arthritis or when cancer metastasises to bone.

Unlike the skin, the internal organs are relatively insensitive to cutting, heat or pinching (Fields, 1987), but twisting and distension are noxious stimuli for hollow viscera such as the gut, the urethra, the gallbladder and urinary bladder. The causes of visceral pain may be summarised as:

- distension;
- spasm or contraction;
- twisting;
- ischaemia (which may be a result of spasm or twisting);
- chemical irritation;
- inflammation.

Certain internal organs, notably the liver and lungs, are reported to be insensitive to pain – that is, pain is not elicited by the normal chemical mechanical or noxious stimuli (Cervero, 1991). However, distension of the liver capsule can cause pain, as well as other symptoms – especially nausea and vomiting – and pleural pain is not uncommon. These observations have important clinical consequences in that many diseases of liver and lungs do not present with pain in the early stage of the disease.

Acute visceral pain is often very intense, dull aching, vaguely localised and accompanied by powerful motor and autonomic reactions, including the abdominal musculature and increased sympathetic outflow. Thus visceral pain may be accompanied by rigidity of the abdominal muscles (guarding) and prominent sympathetic effects – pallor, sweating. Although these reactions are seen accompanying other sorts of pain, a prominent feature of acute visceral pain is the disproportionate response; even small amounts of internal pain are accompanied by dramatic autonomic activity (Cervero, 1991). Furthermore, there is a disproportionate relationship between the amount of internal damage and the pain experienced. A classic example is that of passing a kidney stone. This, in medical terms, is not a serious, life-threatening event; yet it is known to be accompanied by excruciating pain and has been described as one of the most painful events known to humans.

The viscera are not densely innervated – abdominal visceral afferent fibres comprise less than 10% of the total afferent inflow to the spinal cord (Cervero, 1991). Although the nerves are sparse, they can activate a large number of neurones in the spinal cord through functional divergence. This may help to explain why considerable pain may be elicited but the area from which it derives is only poorly identified.

An important aspect of visceral pain is that it can be referred – that is, while the sensation of pain is perceived by the subject in one part of the body, the pathology is in an entirely different tissue. For example, diaphragmatic lesions frequently present with a pain in the shoulder. Visceral pain is frequently referred to a cutaneous site and considerable tenderness may be felt at the site of referral. Referred pain is discussed in more detail below.

3.3 Acute and chronic pain

Pain is often classified by how long it lasts. Thus, temporal descriptions divide pain into acute (short term) and chronic (long term) pain. However, there are important differences between the two, and chronic pain is not just 'long-lasting' acute pain (Table 3.2).

Acute pain is characterised by a well-defined temporal pattern of pain onset. It is accompanied by signs of hyperactivity in the autonomic nervous system, such as sweating and vasoconstriction, that serve to substantiate the patient's reports of pain. Acute pain usually responds to analgesic therapy and treatment of the underlying cause of the pain (Foley, 1993).

By contrast, chronic pain, which is usually defined as that lasting six weeks or more, or associated with a chronic pathological process, is often more difficult to treat. Chronic pain may be enduring pain with an identifiable cause, such as arthritis, or may be harder to explain. In many instances it has an ill-defined temporal onset; patients are often unable to identify when it started. Constant pain produces changes in the CNS which make chronic pain different in nature from acute pain. Adaptation of the autonomic nervous system occurs, so that the patient no longer shows many of the signs that can accompany pain. This can lead an inexperienced observer to doubt the pain's existence. Chronic pain often produces significant changes in personality, life-style and functional ability. Chronic benign pain is discussed in more depth in Chapter 6.

3.4 Chronic pain syndrome

In some patients the effects of chronic pain are so pronounced that their condition is termed 'chronic pain syndrome'. A whole constellation of physical and emotional events are encompassed by this term. Physically, the patient becomes progressively inactive which sets up a vicious circle of ever decreasing mobility. Inactivity causes decreased suppleness in joints, progressive muscle weakness and fatigue. These factors exacerbate the inactivity, increase tiredness and drain the patient's incentive to be active. Inactivity can cause depression and contribute to social withdrawal, which only worsens the condition. Patients show psychological distress, become demoralised and preoccupied with their pain – manifested by excessive use of healthcare facilities and pain medication (excessive is defined in this context as use beyond a level that produces benefit). Personal relationships can become impaired, sometimes affecting the family as a whole. Fear of pain itself can be a factor contributing to the syndrome (McCracken *et al.*, 1992).

Families and/or carers of patients with chronic pain syndrome often express feelings of guilt or inadequacy, since they do not share the pain and can often do little to help break the cycle. Family tensions, arguments and feelings of hopelessness can occur.

A salient feature of the chronic pain syndrome is that it is unrelated to the patient's physical condition. The syndrome may be getting worse, while the patient's physical condition is actually improving. This may be because the behaviour has become learned and reinforced and some psychological intervention may be required to relieve the symptoms. In some situations patients may find that the 'sick role' has brought them benefit either in attention, respite from work or actual compensation. These so-called 'secondary gains' are discussed in more detail in Chapter 4.

Classification of chronic pain

One of the most difficult groups of patients to treat are those who have chronic pain. One of the major factors that has inhibited the advancement of treating chronic pain is the absence of an agreed classification of chronic pain (Turk & Rudy, 1990). Several attempts have been made to produce systems for classifiying chronic pain, but perhaps the most comprehensive is the IASP (International Association for the Study of Pain) taxonomy of chronic pain syndromes (Mersky, 1986), which was revised in 1994 (Mersky & Bogduk, 1994). The IASP system is based on the assignment of patients to predetermined groups based on the match of symptom characteristics. The symptoms are rated along five dimesions or axes, namely:

- body region where the pain exists;
- the body system where abnormal functioning is producing the pain;
- the temporal characteristics of the pain;
- patterns of occurrence (onset, intensity and duration);
- presumed aetiology of the pain.

Each category is rated on a scale from 0 to 8 or 9. This finally gives a five-digit code which classifies the pain. For example, a patient with carpel tunnel syndrome might be classified 204.X6. According to the classification system the digit 2 indicates that the body region is in the upper shoulder and upper limbs; the second digit indicates that the relevant system is the nervous system; the third digit shows that the patient reported pain and that the pain occurred irregularly; the X following the decimal point indicates that the intensity and time of onset will vary with each patient; and the last digit denotes that the presumed aetiology is degenerative or mechanical (Turk & Rudy, 1987a).

The reliability of this system has been established (Turk & Rudy, 1987a). Since the presence of chronic pain can produce behavioural and psychological changes in the patient these authors have also proposed that an appropriate strategy to classify chronic pain patients might consist of the integration of medical-physical, psychosocial, and behavioural data (Turk & Rudy, 1987b; Jamison *et al.*, 1994).

3.5 Referred pain

Pain elicited from the skin is easy to localise, especially in the areas which contain a high density of nociceptive receptors, such as the face and hands. The term 'focal pain' is often used where the sensation is well localised and experienced in the region of the lesion.

By contrast, pain from deeper structures is harder to localise; it is diffuse, spread over a wide area and difficult to pinpoint. Pain is usually felt in a larger area than the tissue affected, and sometimes no definite place can be identified as the painful area. For example, in the early stages of appendicitis pain is felt diffusely over the entire abdomen.

Localisation of visceral pain and, to a lesser extent, musculoskeletal pain is further confounded by the phenomenon of referred pain. This is defined as pain felt in a different area from the site of the pathology. Visceral pain is most commonly referred to a cutaneous site and the underlying muscles whereas musculoskeletal pain is referred to skin and/or other musculoskeletal structures.

When pain is referred the affected area of skin becomes hypersensitive and has definite margins, with the muscles becoming tender. The zones of cutaneous hypersensitivity and muscle tenderness are similar (but not invariable) among patients. This is because the boundaries of the zones of cutaneous hypersensitivity correspond to areas innervated by nerves arising from defined spinal segments. These areas are called dermatomes (Figures 3.3 and 3.4).

Dermatomes are best understood if we look at how the body develops from the embryo. By 3 weeks the embryo consists of a notochord which is the central framework of the spine and mesodermal cells that parallel the notochord and differentiate into three parts: skin (*dermatome*), muscle, tendon and ligaments (*myotome*) and bone (*sclerotome*). The corresponding spinal nerve for each segment develops and innervates these components of the segment. As the skin, muscle and bone develop and migrate to their final location in the body, the cells of each segment retain their corresponding nerve supply. Thus a given afferent nerve that enters the dorsal root seems to be comprised of nerves that come from a widespread area of the body, but the tissues innervated were all from the same embryonic origin.

Dermatomes are labelled according to the nerve that supplies them. The nerves are prefixed C, T, L or S corresponding to the anatomical region of the spinal cord which these nerves enter. Thus C stands for cervical nerves, T for thoracic nerves, L for lumbar nerves and S for sacral nerves. Within each anatomical region the nerves are numbered starting at 1, closest to the head. There are 8 cranial nerves, 12 thoracic nerves, 5 lumbar nerves and 3 sacral nerves.

The viscera are also supplied by nerves which have a defined pathway and are associated with a particular dorsal root. Since the innervation of the viscera and the innervation of the corresponding dermatome converge at the same segment of the spinal cord (i.e. had the same origin in the embryo), there is the possibility that neural inputs are mis-interpreted or incorrectly ascribed by the brain.

There are several ways in which this could happen. If information from the skin and from an internal organ is arriving at the same dorsal horn neurone, this neurone could incorrectly interpret which nerve fibre has sent the pain message (Figure 3.5a). If the afferent nerve innervating a

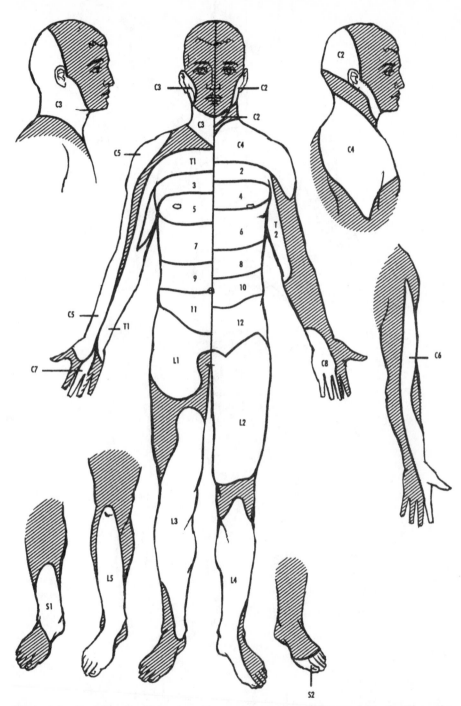

Figure 3.3 Dermatomes, front view. These represent areas of innervation that share the same embryonic origins (see text). Reproduced from Borenstein, D.G. & Wiesel, S.W. (1989) *Low Back Pain*, p. 31, with kind permission of W.B. Saunders Company.

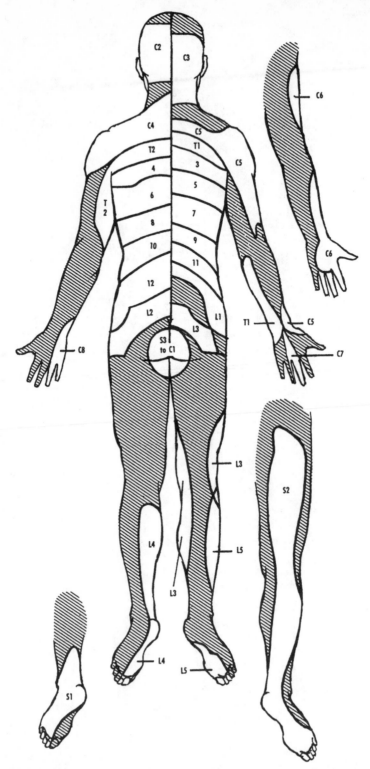

Figure 3.4 Dermatomes, back view. Reproduced from Borenstein, D.G. & Wiesel, S.W. (1989) *Low Back Pain*, p. 32, with kind permission of W.B. Saunders Company.

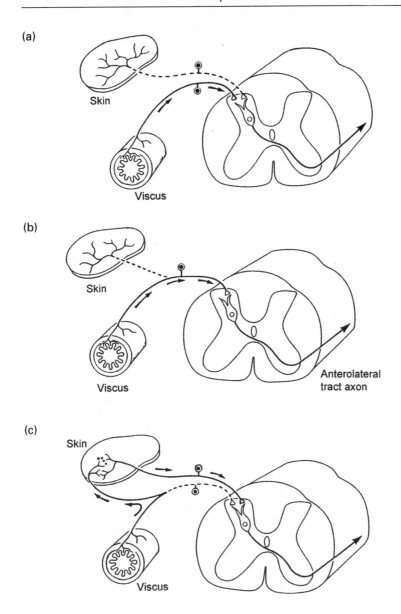

Figure 3.5 Mechanisms of referred pain. Modified from Fields, H.L. (1987) *Pain*.

viscus is branched to supply both the viscus and the more superficial site, then again the brain may misinterpret the information (Figure 3.5b). In a branched pathway nociceptive impulses from the viscus could anti-dromically (in the opposite direction to usual) stimulate the superficial structure (Figure 3.5c). If the more superficial structure is a muscle group, such antidromic activation can cause the muscles to go into spasm which gives rise to pain. If the superficial structure is a muscle group, then such activation can cause muscle spasm which gives rise to pain.

Nociceptors arising in the superficial tissue would then be activated, so that the brain would be interpreting the impulses correctly but the origin of the input would not be the superficial tissue.

It is likely that several mechanisms contribute to referred pain. In some instances local anaesthetic injected at the site of the referred pain will alleviate the condition. This shows that the mislocalisation of pain is due to a process in the CNS, since there is no anaesthetic-sensitive nociceptive input from the site at which the pain is felt. In other cases this procedure has no effect on the referred pain.

Referred pain is a 'one-way' system from deeper to more superficial structures – for example, a cut on the hand will not be referred to the abdomen! Some of the more common sites of referred pain are shown in Figure 3.6.

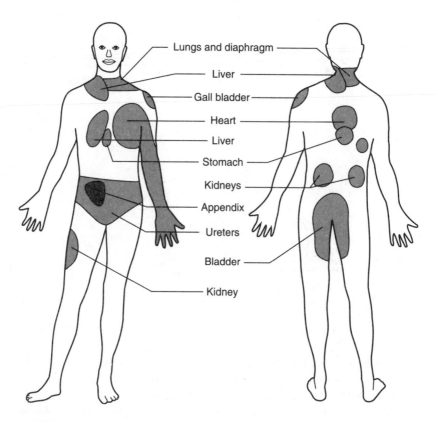

Figure 3.6   Anterior and posterior views showing the common sites where pain is referred from the viscera.

3.6 Radicular pain

Radicular pain is caused by damage to a nerve root. Since a nerve root supplies a large area of tissue, the myotome and dermatome (see Figures 3.3. and 3.4), the pain may be felt anywhere in the distribution of that nerve root. Thus the pain may seem to be in the skin, but is actually due to damage of a much deeper structure. It should not be confused with referred pain, where the source of pain may be any structure, not just a nerve root.

Metastases in the spinal cord can be a source of radicular pain if they compress the nerve root. Radicular pain can also be caused by other types of damage to the nerve root such as that caused by viruses, especially herpes (see section 3.15).

3.7 Breakthrough or incident pain

Patients who have long-term pain problems may have a 'baseline' level of pain which is controlled with suitable medication and/or non-pharmacological techniques. However these patients may also have intermittent, transient periods of more intense pain which 'breaks through' the 'baseline' level of persistent discomfort. These events have a variety of causes, some of the commonest being:

- movement;
- pressure;
- constipation;
- flatulence;
- low plasma levels of analgesics.

The term 'breakthough pain' is also used to refer to the situation where analgesia is inadequate for the degree of pain.

Some events which are likely to cause pain may be anticipated, such as movement or pressure near an affected part of the body. This is also sometimes termed 'incident pain'. This term can also denote pain produced by precipitating factors over which the patient has no control, such as flatulence (Portenoy & Hagen, 1990). Furthermore, incident pain can be caused by some treatments, such as injections or infusions (also called intervention pain) and by some drugs, diagnostic techniques or by the after-effects of radiation. In these cases it may be useful to anticipate the pain and provide extra analgesic cover before the procedure is carried out.

Decreasing plasma levels of analgesics as the time for the next dose is approached can be responsible for breakthrough pain, although appropriate and careful use of analgesics can circumvent this problem.

Table 3.2 The major types of clinical pain.

Type of pain	Cause and major features
Nociceptive	Pain produced by an identifiable stimulus.
Pathological	Pain felt due to activity in the nociceptive pathway which may be due to an identifiable stimulus or due to disruption of normal sensory mechanisms. Pain is usually disproportionate to the causative factors. It may be inappropriate and often outlasts the original trauma.
Neuropathic pain	See Table 3.1.
Somatic	Pain of the somatic tissue – muscle, fascia, tendons. Usually dull aching pain.
Cutaneous	Pain of the skin, usually sharp and well localised.
Visceral pain	Pain of the internal organs, diffuse and difficult to localise. Very intense, dull aching.
Acute pain	Pain of short duration. Usually nociceptive pain.
Chronic pain	Long-lasting pain or pain disproportionate to the cause. It may be pathological pain associated with changes in the CNS or may be due to a constant stimulus.
Chronic pain syndrome	Syndrome induced by long-term pain where pain and responses to the pain are not well correlated with the underlying condition. Changes in personality, behaviour and functional ability occur.
Referred pain	Pain felt in a different area to the source of the pain. Usually referred from organs or deep tissue to muscles and skin.
Radicular pain	Pain caused by damage to a nerve root and felt in the area of distribution of that root.
Breakthrough or incident pain	Short period of sharper or more intense pain that 'breaks through' a background or constant discomfort or pain. Caused by movement, pressure or treatment interventions.
Phantom limb pain	Sensation of pain where a limb has been amputated.
Intractable pain	Pain unrelieved by normal analgesia.
Idiopathic pain	Pain which is excessive for the underlying cause.

3.8 Intractable pain

Intractable pain is a term for pain which is unrelieved despite the use of a wide variety of treatments. There is no one cause of intractable pain and it can derive from many different pathologies. Chronic pain may become intractable, and there is considerable overlap in these terms.

3.9 Idiopathic pain

Idiopathic pain is the term for pain which appears to be excessive for its underlying organic cause. Sometimes the term is used for pain which has no identifiable origin. Thus, it is not a definition of the pathology of the pain. Some patients with idiopathic pain also present with affective and behavioural disturbances which may suggest a psychiatric condition. The term idiopathic pain may be used just to give the pain a label, when really the problem is inadequate clinical diagnosis. Pain should therefore be thoroughly investigated by specialist units before it can truly be said to have no identifiable origin.

The major features of these different types of pain are summarised in Table 3.2.

Part 2: Common clinical conditions associated with severe or prolonged pain

It is impossible to discuss here all the clinical conditions that cause pain. This section covers the more pertinent information about the most frequently encountered clinical conditions that are associated with severe, prolonged or constant pain. Nurses will undoubtedly encounter many more painful conditions than we have space to consider.

3.10 Cancer pain

The cancer patient is a potential victim of a large number of causes of pain. The tumour itself may cause pain, metastases from the primary tumour can cause pain in another area of the body, diagnostic interventions and cancer treatments are sometimes a source of pain or associated with post-treatment syndromes that cause discomfort or are painful. Where tumours are accessible, they may be surgically removed. Thus the cancer patient has to contend with the pain of surgery, which may then be closely followed by adjuvant chemotherapy or radiotherapy.

Some of these are predictable, transient pains; others become long-term problems. Even where the prognosis is good the almost universal fear of cancer also produces psychological or emotional pain and, for patients with terminal illness, the problems are even greater. Cancer pain, therefore, presents probably one of the greatest challenges to nurses, even though the number of patients affected may be less than that seen in other conditions. The amount of pain experienced by cancer patients will vary greatly with the site of the primary tumour. Figure 3.7 gives a summary of the incidence of pain seen in patients with different types of cancers.

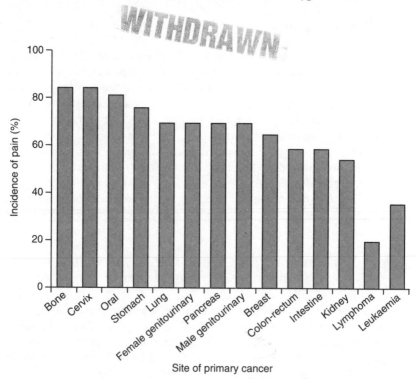

Site of primary cancer

Figure 3.7   Incidence of pain from different cancers. Reproduced from Hanks, G. (1985) Pain control in cancer patients. *Cancer Topics*, **5**, 54–56, with kind permission of Media Medica Publishers Ltd.

Direct tumour involvement

The most common cause of pain in cancer is that associated with direct tumour involvement. Metastatic bone disease, hollow viscus involvement and nerve compression or infiltration are the commonest sources of pain in 78% of cancer inpatients and 62% of problems in outpatients (Foley, 1993). Of these bone tumours are the most predominant cause of pain.

We have already discussed how various mechanisms act to produce pain. The mechanisms are no different in cancer. As neoplastic cells grow, they can directly activate nociceptors mechanically or by releasing agents which affect chemoreceptors. Neoplastic cells can cause local inflammation, releasing inflammatory mediators which activate nociceptors or produce mechanical distortion of receptors.

Tumours can cause direct damage to nerves and can also distort or compress neural tissue, giving rise to acute pain which may be followed by neuropathic pain. An enlarging tissue mass can cause distension of tissue and stimulation of mechanical receptors. Distension of the viscera, such as the liver capsule, or the periosteum of bone is particularly painful.

Radiotherapy or chemotherapy can cause immunosupression which makes a debilitated patient more susceptible to bacterial, viral or fungal infections. Such infections are a source of direct pain or may cause nerve damage leaving the patient with neuropathic pain, as is seen in postherpetic neuralgia.

Bone pain

Bone metastases are the most common cause of chronic pain in advanced cancer. Tumour involvement of bone can cause pain by direct involvement of bone and activation of local nociceptors or by compression of adjacent nerves, soft tissue or vascular structures (Payne & Gonzalez, 1993). The periosteum is particularly sensitive. Tumour metastases of bone are associated with bone destruction and new bone formation. Prostaglandins are important in these changes in bone metabolism and are known to sensitise nociceptors and produce hyperalgesia (Ferriera *et al.*, 1988).

Any tumour type may be complicated by painful bony lesions, but it is cancers of the lung, breast and prostate that most frequently metastasise to bone. The vertebrae are common sites of bony metastases, although any bone can be involved. It is usual for bony metastases to occur in multiple sites, although patients with multiple metastases typically report pain from only a few of these sites (Cherny & Portenoy, 1994). What converts a painless lesion to a painful one is unknown; but when it occurs, the pain is often described as having a 'gnawing' quality. Pain due to a metastatic tumour must be distinguished from other causes of bone pain such as fractures or focal osteonecrosis (a local area of bone damage and necrosis not due to metastases).

There are other problems associated with bony metastases. For example, the pain produced is exacerbated by movement and will often cause patients to become immobile. This immobility can increase resorbtion of bone and elevate plasma calcium levels. High plasma calcium causes nausea and vomiting. Bony metastases also increase the risk of fractures.

Prompt treatment of such conditions may avoid compression of neural structures. This is an important consideration where spinal metastases are present since compression of nerve roots can give radicular pain, and spinal cord compression is a neurological emergency.

Pain syndromes of the viscera

Tumour infiltration of a hollow viscus is the second most common cause of pain in cancer. Such involvement may also involve the pleura or peritoneum, which are more sensitive to pain than some internal organs. Peritoneal carcinomatosis occurs through the spread of abdominal tumours; extra-abdominal tumour cells do not tend to invade the peritoneum. Carcinomatosis can cause several painful conditions: peritoneal inflammation, mesenteric tethering or malignant adhesions.

Pain arising from the viscera may involve recruitment of several different mechanisms which produce pain and can involve mixed neuropathic and nociceptive mechanisms.

Pain sensitive structures in the abdomen include the liver capsule, blood vessels and biliary tract. Referred pain from these organs may be experienced in the shoulder or right scapula. The pain, which is dull and aching, may be exacerbated by movement or pressure in the abdomen (such as constipation) and deep inspiration.

Chronic abdominal obstruction occurs in patients with pelvic or abdominal cancers. The pain is due to smooth muscle contractions, ischaemia in certain areas and distortion or tension in the mesentery. Nerve involvement can also occur. Continuous and colicky pains occur and these can be referred. Vomiting, anorexia and constipation are important symptoms associated with the obstruction.

Tumours of the colon or rectum, female reproductive system and genitourinary system are most commonly responsible for perineal pain. The pain, which is typically constant and aching, is often aggravated by sitting or standing and may be associated with tenesmus or bladder spasm.

Ureteric obstruction is caused by tumour compression or infiltration of the ureter. Ureteric obstruction may be accompanied by pylonephritis which presents with features of sepsis, loin pain and decreased urine flow.

Tumour invasion of the musculature of the deep pelvis can cause a painful myalgia. This is typically a constant ache or heaviness that is exacerbated with upright posture.

Tumours associated with neural tissue

Tumour infiltration of nerves is the third most common cause of pain from direct tumour involvement.

Neuropathic pain may be produced by nerve compression by the tumour, infiltration of the nerve by tumour cells, or a combination of both. This can cause a constant discharge in the nociceptive pathway and a consequent chronic pain. Such pain occurs in 10–15% of advanced cancers (Kenner, 1994).

Tumours of the brain, however, tend not to be painful since there are no sensory nerves within the brain itself. Nevertheless, where the presence of a tumour raises intracranial pressure, then headaches may occur.

3.11 Chronic cancer pain

Cancer patients may have chronic pain which should not be confused with the chronic pain syndrome discussed above. Chronic pain in cancer usually has an insidious onset and is variable in its progression. The pain is related to the patient's physical condition in a way that it is not in the chronic pain syndrome and the patient usually responds appropriately to the changing pain profile. So, the patient's pain may increase as the tumour grows and recede as treatment reduces the tumour. The patient may still show affective disturbances, such as anxiety, sleep disturbances, depression, anorexia and so on, but this will not be so disproportionate to the patient's physical condition. Chronic cancer pain is usually caused by the disease itself, the diagnostic and therapeutic interventions and by the side effects of treatment.

3.12 Postoperative pain

There are various factors involved in surgery that affect the physiological events of pain, as any surgical procedure presents an enormous insult to nociceptive pathways. There will be a phenomenal barrage of afferent information being relayed to the CNS. As discussed in Chapter 2 there is a certain amount of plasticity inherent in peripheral nociceptive pathways. High levels of stimulation can cause changes that result in ·a hyperexcitability of the system with the result that pain will be much greater or elicited more readily.

Anaesthesia is a complex topic but at the simplest level there are basically two main ways of inducing anaesthesia for surgery: general anaesthetic or regional (local) anaesthetic. The different properties of anaesthetics can be exploited to prevent the hyperexcitability caused by surgery from developing.

General anaesthesia techniques have been developed to provide the smallest dose of anaesthetic consistent with the patient's comfort and safety while using paralysing agents to produce immobility. In this situation the massive afferent barrage produced by the surgery reaches the spinal cord and brain. Under regional anaesthesia transmission in the anaesthetised nerve is prevented, and the spinal cord does not receive afferent signals from the surgery (Wall, 1988). Thus local anaesthesia prevents pain-induced changes from occurring in the nociceptive pathways. Similarly, small doses of opioid medication administered before the stimulus occurs can suppress hyperexcitability, whereas much larger doses of opioid are required to achieve the same response once hyperexcitability has been established by the surgical procedure (Wall, 1988; McQuay & Dickenson, 1990).

These observations underpin the clinical practice of giving opioids preoperatively and using local anaesthetic infiltration of the incision site, even when surgery is performed under general anaesthesia. The effects are neatly demonstrated by the results of McQuay *et al.* (1988). This large study looked retrospectively at the time at which patients, grouped according to anaesthetic and premedication, first requested analgesic (Table 3.3).

Table 3.3 Time to requirement of analgesia post surgery. From McQuay and Dickenson (1988).

Patient group	Time to first analgesic (hours) (figures read from graph)
No local anaesthetic No opiate premedication	2
No local anaesthetic Opiate premedication	5.5
Local anaesthetic No opiate premedication	8
Local anaesthetic Opiate premedication	10

Postsurgical pain may stem from conditions associated with the surgery, rather than the surgery itself. For example, anaesthesia can cause gastric stasis, which accompanied by the distension of flatus can be extremely painful. When gas has been used to distend the abdomen, for example during laparoscopy, then the pressure on the diaphragm can cause pain which is referred to the shoulders. Patients may be distressed and confused to find pain in the shoulder after an abdominal procedure.

Certain types of surgery are associated with specific postsurgical pain syndromes. Phantom limb pain and stump pain have been addressed in the first section of this chapter. When assessing postsurgical pain, it is important to differentiate between pain due to surgery and pain due to the disease process. Time of onset is a critical factor in making this assessment.

3.13 Herpetic and postherpetic neuralgia

Viral infections can be a source of pain both during the active phase of infection and post infection. These problems are most often seen with infection by viruses of the herpes family, which tends to rest dormant in nerves. The herpes virus most usually associated with pain is varicella zoster virus (VZV). A primary infection causes chicken pox; a secondary infection produces shingles, involving a posterior root nerve. Since there is nerve involvement, the patient can develop herpetic neuralgia or be left, after an infection, with postherpetic neuralgia.

Anyone can be susceptible to viral infection, but these are obviously more common in debilitated patients, especially those who are immuno-suppressed – either because of disease or because of taking immuno-suppressive medication. Cancer patients have about five times the number of VZV infections as the normal population, and disseminated infection occurs twice as often in patients with active tumours compared with those in remission (Rusthoven *et al.*, 1988). During periods of active VZV infection, acyclovir has been found to be effective in preventing dis-semination of the virus and in diminishing the pain of acute herpetic neuralgia.

Postherpetic neuralgia may follow VZV. It is 2-3 times more frequent in the cancer population than in the general population. The pain is char-acterised by continuous aching, itching, and burning overlaid with par-oxysms of shooting, burning pain. Allodynia and hyperpathia are common. Amitryptiline has been successful in controlling post-herpetic pain, and topical capsaicin has produced transient improvement (Watson *et al.*, 1988). Carbamazepine is useful to control lancinating pain, and neuroleptics, anticonvulsants and anaesthetic approaches have been used. Postherpetic neuralgia may also be treated by sympathetic blockade.

3.14 Anginal pain

Angina pectoris is the pain associated with transient myocardial ischaemia. It describes a syndrome rather than a disease and occurs because the oxygen demands of the cardiac muscles exceed the oxygen supply so that myocardial ischaemia results. Factors which can increase the oxygen demand of the tissue include any which increase the ventricular preload, such as exercise, anaemia or hyperthyroidism, or additional afterload such as that produced by hypertension, aortic stenosis or obstructive cardiomyopathy. Rarely, angina is produced by coronary artery spasm.

Angina is usually experienced as a sense of oppression or tightness in the middle of the chest often described 'like a band round the chest'. Patients typically place a clenched fist on the sternum when describing the pain. It is usually induced by exertion, especially outdoor pursuits or anxiety. Angina is likely to be worse when walking against a wind, uphill, on a cold day and after meals.

Pain is often accompanied by discomfort in the left arm, wrist and fingers of the left hand. The patients often refers to the limb as 'useless'. Less often the pain may be epigastric or intrascapular or may radiate to the neck and jaw without reference to the chest. Rest or medication with amyl trinitrate brings rapid relief.

3.15 Trigeminal neuralgia

Trigeminal neuralgia, or tic douloureux, is characterised by paroxysmal and sharp pain in the distribution of the fifth cranial nerve, that is, along the jaw and across the cheek. The pain does not usually involve the eye, although there is an optic division of the nerve. Each paroxysm of pain lasts only seconds, but several attacks in rapid succession may give the impression of lasting pain. Stabbing pain is frequently interspersed with dull aching pain. Pain is precipitated by touching 'trigger points' which may occur when chewing, talking, washing the face or often when a cold wind blows on the face. Paroxysmal pain may last days or weeks with periods of remission in between. As the disease progresses the periods of remission may become shorter. Trigeminal neuralgia is more prevalent in older patients.

Trigeminal neuralgia is treated with carbamazepine, or in more severe cases trigeminal nerve block may be produced with injections of anaesthetics or cryoanalgesia.

3.16 Arthritis

There is a heterogeneous group of disorders of the joints and bones which are associated with pain and some stiffness in the musculosketal system. These rheumatic diseases form a huge branch of medicine and cannot be covered in any detail here. Two of the more common of these conditions are osteoarthritis and rheumatoid arthritis. Both are long-term, chronic conditions associated with joint pain and increasing disability. The difference between the two types is that rheumatoid arthritis is an inflammatory condition, which may be an autoimmune condition, whereas osteoarthritis is primarily a degenerative disease causing destruction of cartilage. Rheumatoid arthritis can exist as a disease on its own, or it often occurs as a complication of other diseases; many bacterial and fungal infections can be complicated by the development of an arthritic condition.

Rheumatoid arthritis

Rheumatoid arthritis affects women more than men and is more prevalent in older people. The incidence of 1.8% of adult females rises to over 5% of females over 65 years old. It usually has a slow insidious onset, characterised by aches, pains and stiffness, but in 10–20% of cases it appears suddenly over the course of a day (Jayson & Grennan, 1987). Any joint may be affected but typically arthritis is symmetrical and affects one of more of the joints of the wrists, fingers, feet, ankles, knees, and cervical spine. Shoulders, elbows and hips are less commonly affected.

Actively inflamed joints are stiff and painful, particularly on movement. As discussed previously, any inflammation will cause pain. In addition effusions occur and the resultant swelling causes distortion of the joint and pain. Cartilage itself does not contain nociceptors and so is not the site of the pain, but damage or destruction of the cartilage exposes the highly sensitive periosteum which is certainly a source of pain. Osteoporosis can occur and this is associated with prostaglandin activity which causes pain. Experimental systems have shown that during the inflammatory phase of the disease many silent nociceptors are recruited (Grigg *et al.*, 1986). Studies have shown that previously silent afferents develop ongoing activity, giving background pain, and discharge vigorously during ordinary movements. Significantly, arthritic joints display enhanced receptive fields that could not be detected in the healthy joint (McMahon & Koltzenburg, 1990).

Any changes in the joint may cause the patient to move awkwardly and this can place undue strain on nearby muscle groups. As the disease progresses, cartilage, bone and ligament damage become increasingly pronounced to produce the typical deformities seen in long-term destructive rheumatoid arthritis. Rheumatoid arthritis is reviewed in greater depth by Akil and Amos (1995).

Osteoarthritis

Osteoarthritis is very common, affecting about 10% of all adults (Dieppe, 1987). As with rheumatoid arthritis, it is more prevalent in females. The condition is characterised by destruction of cartilage with overgrowth and remodelling of the underlying bone. Basically a disturbance occurs between the stresses applied to a joint and its capacity to withstand them and the joint 'fails' or is incapacitated. It is a multifactorial condition of unknown aetiology, although certain factors have been identified as contributory. There is a genetic predisposition to arthritis, and ageing of the connective tissue has been implicated, as has abnormal joint loading, biochemical abnormalities of the cartilage and previous inflammatory joint disease. Mechanical stress can cause osteoarthritis, but only if abnormal and repetitive. Normal joint use, even to excess as in some sports, does not in itself cause osteoarthritis.

Apart from the lack of an inflammatory response, the sources of pain in osteoarthritis are the same as for rheumatoid arthritis: exposure of the periosteum due to destruction of the cartilage and destruction of bone with prostaglandin involvement.

The mainstay of treatment for all arthritic conditions are the non-steroidal anti-inflammatory drugs (NSAID), which are discussed in detail in Chapter 7. Osteoarthritis is reviewed by Jones and Doherty (1995).

3.17 Migraine

Migraine is a disorder of usually recurrent severe headaches, often accompanied by certain neurological disturbances. In common migraine the pain of the headache develops slowly, sometimes mounting to a throbbing pain that is exacerbated by movement or noise. It is usually, but not invariably, unilateral and accompanied by nausea and vomiting and photophobia. Vomiting often brings relief from the attack.

Classical migraine is comparatively rare. The attack is preceded by a visual disturbance that consists of an area of blindness surrounded by a sparkling or shimmering halo – the so-called aura – that spreads to affect up to half the visual field of each eye, but resolves within half an hour. It is followed by an intense unilateral headache, nausea and/or vomiting.

Migraine occurs in at least 10% of the population and is three times more common in women than men. Migraine can affect children as young as three years old; 60% of sufferers have their first attack before the age of 20 years. It is extremely rare for migraine to first appear after the age of 50.

Migraine runs in families and can be precipitated by a number of factors, as can any tension headache. The most common causes are stress and mental tension, such as anger, worry, excitement, depression, over-exertion, etc. (Rasmussen, 1993). Certain foods (notably chocolate, cheese, red wine and fried foods) are also suspected to be culprits, although this is not universally agreed. Other common precipitating factors are alcohol, weather changes and menstruation (Rasmussen, 1993).

Female hormones seem to be related to the occurrence of migraine, for not only is the incidence higher in women, especially around the time of menstruation, but migraine often has its onset during pregnancy (especially migraine with aura) and can be exacerbated by oral contraceptives (Mazal, 1978).

Migraine occurs in two phases: the first is constriction of the intracranial arteries causing ischaemia in the brain and the prodromal signs followed by dilatation of the extracranial arteries causing the throbbing headache. It starts with a spreading area of decreased blood flow across the cortex forwards from the temporal lobe (Lauritzen & Olesen, 1984). This hypoperfusion outlasts the early symptoms and spreads well into the headache phase. Both vascular actions are thought to be due to serotonin. It has long been known that excretion of the main metabolite of serotonin,

5-HIAA (5-hydroxyindole acetic acid), is vastly increased during a migraine attack accompanied by a fall in the platelet concentration of this compound. However, it cannot be assumed that all the serotonin is platelet derived, and the release of intracerebral serotonin may also be involved.

Many treatments of migraine involve drugs that act on the serotoninergic system. Since serotonin has complex actions on the cerebral and extracerebral circulation, both serotonin antagonists such as pizotifen, cyproheptadine and methysergide and serotonin agonists such as sumatriptan are effective. (The pharmacology of these drugs is discussed in more detail in Chapter 7.) Interestingly, an age-old remedy for headaches and sickness – the herb feverfew (*Tanacetum partenium*) – contains a group of chemicals, the sesquiterpene lactones, which act on platelets to reduce serotonin release.

3.18 Labour pain

Most women experience intense pain during labour, although labour pain shows an astonishingly high degree of variability among individuals (Melzack, 1984). In biological terms this is a strange phenomenon – why should something that is so important to survival of the species be painful?

Many processes involved in labour and childbirth will give rise to pain. The strong contractions of the abdominal muscles are painful and give rise to a generalised neuroendocrine stress response; the dilatation of the cervix and stretching of the vagina as the baby emerges are powerful stimuli to mechanoreceptors. A detailed discussion of these processes is given by Brownridge (1995).

It has been shown that a woman's pain threshold does in fact increase during the last 16 days of pregnancy (Cogan & Spinnato, 1986), this increase being even more marked during the last 9 days. Discomfort thresholds during the last 9 days before delivery were also higher than in non-pregnant controls. A study in animal models has shown an abrupt rise in pain threshold 1–2 days before parturition (Gintzler, 1980) which was mediated by endorphins. So, perhaps as preparation for the event of childbirth, neurochemical changes occur to increase pain thresholds, maybe by elevating endogenous opiates.

Despite these preparative measures, childbirth is still a painful experience. Using the McGill pain questionnaire, one study (Belanger *et al.*, 1989) has shown that primiparas (first delivery) report more pain than multiparas (second or later delivery) and that labour pain was more painful than many clinical conditions, superseded in pain score only by causalgia or accidental amputation of a digit. However, the duration of these pains is so vastly different that in some ways the comparison is debatable.

Not only was the overall pain score less in multiparous women but fewer reported severe pain (45% compared with 60% of primiparous women) and more had mild pain (25% compared with only 10% of primiparous women). These results were similar to those obtained by Niven and Gijsbers (1984).

Interestingly these results also showed that childbirth training (learned relaxation and breathing techniques) was effective in reducing labour pain, but not dramatically. This is consistent with a previous study which showed that small amounts of relaxation affected pain perception, but this effect did not increase with extensive practice (Cogan, 1978). Various pharmacological and non-pharmacological interventions are available for the relief of labour pain. An important consideration is providing adequate pain relief for the mother without untoward effects on the baby. The most common interventions are relaxation, entonox (gas and air) and epidural anaesthesia. These are discussed in more detail in Chapter 7.

3.19 Burn pain

Exposure to heat stimulates thermal receptors and produces the sensation of burning. Initial sensations are C-fibre and A-fibre mediated, and further A-fibre sensitisation also occurs. Above temperatures of 49°C actual tissue damage occurs. There are three degrees of burn depending on the extent of the damage.

First-degree burns involve only the epidermis or top layer of skin. They heal quickly, but the damaged skin may peel away in a day or two. Sunburn is a common example.

Second-degree burns damage the skin more deeply, causing the formation of blisters. Although the damage extends beyond the epidermis, not all of the dermis of the skin is damaged; and as a result, these burns usually heal without scarring unless they are particularly severe.

Third-degree burns destroy the full thickness of the skin and may expose muscle or bone.

All burns are painful and local burns are accompanied by a surrounding area of mechanical hyperalgesia. It is essential to reduce the heat in the burned tissue as quickly as possible to prevent further damage. Thus burns are placed under cold running water or covered with a cold compress. Second- or third-degree burns covering 10% or more of the body are accompanied by extensive fluid loss which places the patient in a state of shock, with lowered blood pressure and increased pulse. Intravenous fluids are essential.

Burned skin is no longer protective and infection from airborne bacteria, viruses and or fungi present life-threatening complications. Inhalation of smoke in a fire can cause swelling and inflammation of the lungs which can cause suffocation.

3.20 Back pain

Second to the common cold, back pain is the most prevalent affliction of man (Borenstein & Wiesel, 1989). A recent survey of over 3000 subjects aged 25–64 years, randomly selected from a Family Health Service Register, showed an annual incidence of low back pain of 4.7%, with a lifetime prevalence of 59% – over half the population (Hillman *et al.*, 1996). The incidence of low back pain can be influenced by age and occupation; individuals in jobs which involve heavy physical work or lifting being more susceptible to back pains than others (Savage *et al.*, 1997). Back pain sufferers constitute a large proportion of the people receiving benefits for incapacity to work and is associated with a high rate of relapse. A study in Canada revealed that around 20% of individuals absent from work due to back pain relapse in the first six months after return to work (Infante-Rivard *et al.*, 1997).

Back pain has a variety of causes and can often be very difficult to diagnose. This situation is complicated by the fact that the majority of back pains resolve spontaneously; 80–90% of patients are better within a two-month period with or without medical intervention. This information suggesting that many patients will not need any active treatment, must be tempered by the fact that the earlier the intervention, the better the prognosis. Once back pain has lasted six weeks it is likely to become chronic, and at six months there is only a 50% chance of return to work (Ellis, 1995). This presents healthcare professionals with a real dilemma, and emphasises the need for accurate diagnosis in the first instance.

Back pains have a variety of causes which are broadly mechanical, inflammatory or neurological. The major causes of back pain are summarised according to the source of the pain in Table 3.4. The underlying pathology of most of these sources of pain has been covered above. The difficulty of diagnosis will vary with the cause of pain and a precise diagnosis will not be possible in many patients. Some conditions, such as skin disorders, are visible, while vertebral disc lesions will require a thorough neurological examination. Diseases of internal viscera which are causing back pain will need physical examination and perhaps other interventions to enable a diagnosis to be made. Some cancers, notably ovarian and prostate, metastasise to bone, often in the spine giving rise to back pain. The most elusive pains are those of psychogenic origins.

Treatment of back pain will be dependent on an identifiable cause; anti-inflammatory, antispamodics and antibiotic drugs may be used. Where pain is due to cancer (primary or in cases of spinal matastases) radiotherapy or radionuclides are used. Topical NSAIDs can bring relief to muscle strains. Physiotherapy is of major importance in treating back pains and maintaining mobility must be a priority. Back pain sufferers often gain relief from non-invasive techniques such as heat or cold therapy.

Table 3.4 Causes of back pain. Reproduced from Borenstein and Weisel (1989) by permission of W.B. Saunders.

Category	Pathology	Quality of pain	Location	Intensity	Onset and duration	Aggravating and alleviating factors
Superficial somatic	Cellulitis	Sharp	Well localised	Correlates with intensity of nerve stimulation (mild to moderate)	Acute	Intensified by direct contact
	Herpes zoster	Burning			Correlates with status of lesion	Diminished by light touch in adjacent area
Deep somatic (muscles, fascia, periosteum, ligament, joints, vessels, dura)	Muscular strain	Sharp (acute)	Diffuse	Correlates with intensity of nerve stimulation	Acute or chronic	Intensified with movement Diminished with rest
	Arthritis	Dull ache (chronic)	Multiple segments affected			
Bone	Tuberculosis Neoplasm – primary or metastases	Severe tenderness	Multiple segments affected			Systemic signs – weight loss, fever, etc.

Radicular (spinal nerves)	Herniated vertebral disc	Segemental	Low back	Mild to severe	Acute	Intensified with standing, sitting
	Spinal stenosis	Radiating	Afferent distribution of affected nerve root	Correlates with intensity of nerve impingement	Acute	Diminished with bed rest
Visceral referred	Pancreatitis	Deep	Segemental with radiation inside body	Mild to severe	Acute or chronic	Related to factors affecting relevant organ system
	Intestinal disease (numerous)	Boring		Correlates with intensity of nerve stimulation	Acute or chronic	
	Prostatitis Endometriosis Abdominal aneurysm	Colicky Tearing				

A prominent feature of all types of chronic back pain is that it may be accompanied by depression (see also section 3.4). The prevalence of major depression in patients with chronic low back pain is approximately three to four times greater than reported in the general population (Sullivan *et al.*, 1992). For this reason antidepressants deserve serious consideration as an integral component of the pain management programme (Sullivan *et al.*, 1992). A more detailed discussion of pain management programmes in chronic non-malignant pain, such as backpain, is given in Chapter 6.

3.21 Chronic pelvic pain

Chronic pelvic pain (CPP) is a debilitating condition that mainly affects younger, premenopausal, women. CPP is most commonly defined as pain in the pelvic region, which has persisted for more than six months and is not relieved by non-opioid analgesics (Wiener, 1994). The annual incidence of pelvic pain in the UK is estimated as 14 000 with a prevalence of 345 000, costing the Health Service over £182 million (Davies *et al.*, 1992).

Pelvic pain does not always have an identifiable organic cause, and the condition is made more complex since it can have a variety of gynaecological or non-gynaecological causes (Table 3.5), which may not be clearly distinguished. Many female patients with irritable bowel syndrome have

Table 3.5 Causes of chronic pelvic pain. Reproduced from Weiner (1994) with kind permission of *The Practitioner.*

Gynaecological causes
- Chronic pelvic inflammatory disease
- Endometriosis
- Pelvic pain syndrome
- Neoplasm (benign or malignant)
- Residual ovary syndrome
- Uterovaginal prolapse

Non-gynaecological causes
- Gastro-intestinal:
  – irritable bowel syndrome
  – diverticulitis
- Renal:
  – chronic interstitial cystitis
  – caliculi
  – malignancy
- Musculoskeletal:
  – osteoarthritis
  – intervertebral disc prolapse

associated gynaecological symptoms and present to gynaecologists when the underlying problem is gastro-intestinal (Longstreth, 1994). It is important therefore that the cause of the patient's pain is investigated fully.

Symptoms can give clues as to whether the cause of the pain is infection or related to the menstrual cycle. Laparoscopy is often necessary in making a firm diagnosis of the source of CPP, and for a small percentage of patients even laparoscopy cannot reveal the underlying pathology. Such patients are often referred to as having 'pelvic pain syndrome'. Pelvic pain is discussed in more detail in Weiner (1994).

WITHDRAWN

3.22 Treatment-related pain

For some patients the treatment for their condition can also induce pain. Usually this pain is short lived and does not extend beyond the period of treatment. Repeated painful episodes can cloud a patient's view of his or her treatment, affecting morale and compliance with treatment. So, such pain deserves consideration for patient well-being and, since it is often predictable, can be minimised or avoided with some simple forward planning. The aim of the healthcare team must be to demonstrate an awareness of the problem and to manage the pain effectively.

Intravenous, intramuscular and subcutaneous injections

Any injections for administering medication or venepuncture for obtaining a blood sample can be painful. Proper explanation of what is about to happen and attempts to make the patient relax are useful. Local anaesthesia of the injection site is helpful, and the usual technique is to apply EMLA (eutectic mixture of local anaesthetic – see Chapter 7) cream to the injection site some minutes before the procedure.

3.23 Miscellaneous pain problems in bedridden patients

There are a number of problems that affect patients who have to spend prolonged periods in bed. This list is not exhaustive but the most frequently encountered problems are: muscle spasm, constipation, pressure ulcers/bedsores, deep vein thrombosis.

Where patients constantly lie in the same position, or if injury or disease is causing the patient to adopt an abnormal posture, an undue strain can be placed on certain muscles and a long-term muscle pain can develop. These pains are usually localised and aching. They are best treated by identifying the position that brings relief and helping the patient understand the need for resting an overworked muscle group. Massage and physiotherapy can be useful.

Table 3.6 Some pointers to identifying sources of pain. (For back pains see Table 3.4.)

Ask	Consider
Is the pain related to breathing?	Lung infection, emphysema, bronchitis, pleurisy, pulmonary embolism
Is the pain related to eating?	Mouth problems, ulcers, oesophagitis, gastro-intestinal obstruction
Is there joint pain?	Joint inflammation, infection, arthritis, bleeding (haemophiliacs and leukaemics), metastatic disease
Is there a tight band of pain around the chest plus pain in the left arm?	Spinal cord compression angina, myocardial infarction
Is pain related to the bowel?	Constipation; irritable bowel syndrome (IBS), infection, bowel obstruction, excessive flatulence, occlusion of blood flow, peritonitis
With rectal bleeding?	Haemorrhoids; Crohn's disease; colorectal cancer
Is the pain the suprapubic region?	Bladder infection; outflow obstruction; unstable bladder; irritation by tumour
Is the pain in the loin or groin area?	Urinary tract infection; obstruction
Does passive movement exacerbate the pain?	Nerve compression, soft tissue inflammation, pathological fracture, bony metastases
Is pain worse on active movement?	Myofascial pain; skeletal muscle strain or spasm
Is there an identifiable skin lesion?	Trauma; pressure damage; infection; irritation; allergy; skin disease
Are there general skin changes (mottled/glossy)?	Sympathetically maintained pain
Is there a burning or tingling quality to the pain?	Neuropathic pain
Are there unpleasant sensory changes?	Neuropathic pain; sympathetically maintained pain; peripheral nerve damage; postherpetic neuralgia
Are there constitutional changes (weight loss, fever)?	Infection, tumour
Are there signs of CNS involvement?	Spinal cord compression; cranial nerve damage; thalamic pain, meningitis
Does the pain follow a peripheral nerve distribution?	Radicular pain, nerve root compression, referred pain from internal organ

Prolonged periods in bed can cause pressure ulcers or bed sores. These terms describe any area of damage to the skin or underlying tissue caused by direct pressure of shearing forces. Damage can vary in severity from erythema to necrotic ulceration involving muscle, tendon and bone. Direct pressure, such as can be produced by lying in the same position, can cause capillary obstruction and deprive tissue of oxygen. Such ischaemia can cause tissue damage. Shearing occurs when a patient slips down the bed or is dragged up the bed. (Mallett & Bailey, 1996).

The most likely areas for the development of pressure ulcers are the sacral area, coccygeal area, ischial tuberosities or the greater trochanters. Pressure ulcers may be avoided by frequent repositioning of the patient; but when sores develop, pain relief and appropriate wound care is essential. A detailed consideration of the condition is given by Mallett and Bailey (1996). Immobility, especially after surgery, can also give rise to complications such as deep vein thrombosis.

Bed rest or analgesics, especially opioids, are often associated with constipation which may be a painful condition.

Obviously diagnosing any pain is a complex task; the source of some pains remains elusive even to healthcare professionals with many years clinical experience. Table 3.6 suggests a few pointers to identifying pains but is by no means comprehensive.

Summary of Chapter 3

- No universal system for classifying pain exists.
- Neuropathic pain does not require the presence of an identifiable noxious stimulus.
- Unusual activity in the sympathetic nervous system can cause sympathetically maintained pain.
- Damage to the CNS results in central pain.
- Interruption of peripheral nerves causes deafferentation pain; loss of these nerves causes peripheral neuropathies.
- Loss of a limb can leave a residual pain in the stump or the sensation of a phantom limb.
- Pain may be classified according to whether it occurs in the musculoskeletal system, the internal organs or the skin. Referred pain can confuse these definitions.
- Long-term changes mean that chronic pain is not just merely long-lasting acute pain.
- Other types of pain are: radicular, breakthrough, intractable or idiopathic.
- Common conditions causing severe or long-term pain are discussed in detail.

Chapter 4

The Pain Experience

4.1 Introduction

Pain is a fundamental and inevitable form of human suffering, the experience of which is unique to each individual. Eland (1978) described her experience of postherpetic trigeminal neuralgia as a 'living hell'. She says that little by little people are destroyed by chronic intractable pain until they become a shadow of their former selves. Not everyone has such a distressing pain experience. For many mothers the pain of childbirth diminishes greatly and is often forgotten when their new-born baby is placed in their arms. Thus, pain can have a very different meaning for each person.

Many factors are thought to affect a person's perception and tolerance of pain. These include the meaning of the pain, a person's emotional state and the degree to which people feel they are in control of the situation. There is also enormous variation in how each individual will express pain. A person's cultural background, beliefs and attitudes, personality, and gender has a powerful influence on pain expression. In addition, if someone gains some practical, financial or emotional advantage from their pain, they may express it more frequently and in an exaggerated manner. The purpose of this chapter is to explore the nature of the pain experience, and the factors which are thought to influence a person's perception and expression of pain.

4.2 The nature of the pain experience

Over fifty years ago Rene Leriche defined pain as '... the resultant of the conflict between a stimulus and the whole individual' (Leriche, 1939). This definition highlights the fact that pain is not merely a bodily experience; it is a phenomenon which is modulated by physical, psychological, social, cultural and spiritual factors (Cassel, 1982; Mount, 1993). This viewpoint has led some people to question the homogeneity of the word 'pain'. Saunders (1967) has coined the term 'total pain' in order to help people understand the nature of chronic pain in cancer patients (Figure 4.1). The model of total pain draws attention to the many variables which influence a patient's perception and tolerance of pain (Twycross, 1994).

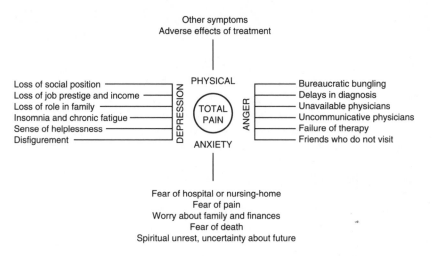

Figure 4.1   The concept of total pain. Reproduced from Twycross, R. (1994) *Pain relief in Advanced Cancer*, p. 28, with kind permission of Churchill Livingstone.

Although this model has been created to explain the nature of pain in patients with advanced cancer, it is of relevance to all forms of pain. This is because pain, regardless of type, does not occur within a vacuum. It occurs in a whole person who has many facets, and if healthcare professionals ignore any one of these facets when caring for the patient in pain, they may contribute significantly to that patient's suffering (Cassel, 1982).

4.3 Pain threshold and tolerance

In relation to pain, 'threshold' can be defined as the lowest limit at which a stimulus becomes perceptible or the highest limit at which a stimulus is bearable (*Oxford English Dictionary*, 1988). Threshold can be measured by applying a stimulus, such as electric shock or heat, and recording when the subject starts to notice a sensation. Four different types of threshold have been demonstrated by Melzack and Wall (1982):

- sensation threshold – the lowest value at which a sensation is perceived;
- pain perception threshold – the lowest level at which the sensation feels painful;
- pain tolerance – the upper limit at which the subject asked for the sensation to be withdrawn;
- encouraged pain tolerance threshold – the level at which the subject can be encouraged to tolerate the sensation.

Thus, pain thresholds can be viewed as both physiological and psychological responses to painful stimuli, with perception being predominantly physiological and tolerance mostly psychological. It is important not to confuse the concepts of tolerance to pain and tolerance to drugs such as opioids (see Chapter 5).

The sensation threshold does not appear to vary considerably between individuals, even though there can be considerable variation in other thresholds. For example, Beecher (1956) found that the analgesic requirement for soldiers wounded in battle was much less than that of civilians with comparable injuries as a result of accidents. He suggested that differences existed because the soldiers viewed their injuries as a means of escape from the battlefield, whereas the civilians viewed their injuries as a threat to their lifestyle. This example and the many others which are reported in the literature, highlight the fact that numerous factors influence pain perception and tolerance. This situation can be exploited to the patient's benefit in clinical practice by mobilising factors which increase the pain perception threshold and by using encouragement to help the patient tolerate pain. The former of these strategies is more appropriate for chronic pain, the latter seems an appropriate strategy for acute pain.

4.4 Factors which influence the perception of pain

A wide range of factors are thought to influence a person's perception and tolerance of pain, including the meaning of the pain, cultural background, religion, sense of control over pain, gender and emotions such as anxiety and depression.

Meaning of the pain

Pain can have a range of different meanings for people. Pain serves quite a useful purpose when it draws attention to injury or illness. Many pains pass very quickly and have a limited impact on the person's life. For example, if you fall and bruise your knee, you know the reason for the pain and that it will go away eventually, whereas with chronic pain the situation is less straightforward. Pain has stopped serving any useful purpose, and it is impossible to say how long it will persist, indeed for many patients it may persist for the rest of their lives. For cancer patients, increasing levels of pain may be equated with disease progression and be viewed as a metaphor for impending death by both patient and family (Spiegel & Bloom, 1983a; Garro, 1990; Ferrell *et al*, 1991; Ferrell & Dean, 1995). Such an interpretation may result in patients experiencing more pain since there is evidence that severity of pain is positively associated with how people interpret the significance of their pain. For example, Spiegel and Bloom (1983) found a significant correlation between the belief that pain was indicative of worsening disease and reports of more severe pain.

The pain of childbirth is often viewed by women as being different to other types of pain. It has a very special meaning since it results in the birth of a child and consequently, is seen in a more positive light. In a small study of psychological factors associated with pain in labour reported by Moore (1997), many of the women had a very positive attitude towards labour pain. The pain was 'worth the discomfort', 'a wonderful thing' and 'had meaning'. Such attitudes may be fostered by a partner who is supportive throughout pregnancy and labour and have been shown to reduce pain during labour (Bonica, 1994). By contrast, an ambivalent or negative attitude towards the pregnancy may result in an increase in pain perception during labour.

The meaning a person has for a given illness is often closely linked with the coping strategies which are adopted to cope with the burdens of that illness (Lipowski, 1970). This researcher found that the meaning of illness in North American culture can be classified as challenge; enemy; punishment; weakness; relief; strategy; loss; value.

A number of nurse researchers have found that Lipowski's categories are represented in the meaning patients attributed to their pain (Copp, 1974; Barkwell, 1991; Ferrell & Dean, 1995). It is clear that patients derive a range of different meanings from their pain experience. Ferrell and Dean (1995) suggest that an important intervention for those who construe pain in a negative way is to facilitate them to derive a more positive meaning for their pain. For instance, if patients believe that their pain cannot be controlled, then it should be demonstrated that the pain can be relieved. This suggestion is supported by the findings of Arathuzik's (1991) study of women with metastatic breast cancer, which demonstrated that patients who perceive their pain as threatening or harmful find it difficult to accept pain and do not think they can live with it. This reaction is associated with a higher reported pain intensity. Conversely, patients who viewed their pain in a more positive light experienced less emotional distress from their pain and were able to devise a range of strategies to deal with pain. This reaction was associated with less reported pain intensity.

Cultural background

A person's cultural background is thought to influence the meaning that person will attribute to a pain experience. A number of writers would suggest that Western culture has not always attributed the same meaning and emotional significance to the experience of pain (Illich, 1976; Menges, 1984). They argue that over the last century Western cultures have become medicalised and, as a result, people have become less tolerant of pain and have greater expectations about 'curing' it, an expectation which, for some pains, is far beyond the capability of modern medicine (Bendelow & Williams, 1995). As a result Western society places a high value on the use of analgesics and sophisticated drug delivery devices to ameliorate pain. By contrast, during the last century, it was routine for procedures to be carried out without the aid of analgesics, despite the fact that such substances were available (albeit to a lesser extent than today).

There are a number of reasons why these unrealistic expectations have emerged. In years gone by pain was viewed as a natural and inevitable part of life and therefore was accepted as normal. Pain was omnipresent, which meant that there was no frame of reference for people to view it as abnormal (Zola, 1975). The more successful we are at controlling pain, the less omnipresent pain becomes and the greater the tendency to view it as an abnormal and unnatural part of life. Thus, contemporary Western society does not find pain to be acceptable – it is an abnormality that needs to be controlled. This attitude is very well illustrated in a study by Kodiath and Kodiath (1992) who compared the chronic benign pain experience of people from a Western (American) and Eastern (Indian) culture. They found that even though the pain condition was the same, two completely different phenomena emerged. Indians found meaning in their pain, whereas Americans searched for a way to eliminate their pain. This resulted in significantly different consequences for the two cultures. The authors concluded that there is a link between the degree of suffering and the meaning of pain for a person and that the ability to find meaning in a particular situation may be culturally determined.

Religious beliefs

Some people believe that pain has positive qualities because it provides a means of spiritual and moral atonement. This belief is deeply rooted and legitimised by many of the world's most successful religions (Kotarba, 1983; Wall & Jones, 1991). For centuries martyrs and saints faced cruel and painful deaths because they refused to renounce their faiths. Such acts have been immortalised and highly praised by the various organised religions, particularly the Christian churches. The legitimisation and rationalisation of suffering in this life has led some people to believe that self-infliction of pain or the endurance of pain associated with a disease may in some way raise their moral stature, thereby guaranteeing a more swift entry to the afterlife, a place free from all pain and suffering. Pain and suffering are often seen to be the will of God, a means by which God tests loyalty, purifies, and provides opportunity for redemption. These beliefs often enable people to accept pain with great equanimity since they foster a great sense of hope.

Religious beliefs may also cause pain to be seen in a more negative light. Some patients will view pain as a punishment for sins of the past as a form of divine retribution. This can be very frightening for terminally ill patients who believe that they are soon to meet their 'Maker', especially if they view God as being unforgiving. Such beliefs may have been reinforced over a lifetime of religious indoctrination, are therefore extremely difficult to dispel, and can contribute greatly to the patient's perception of pain.

Sense of control

Perceived control over an event is an important determinant of response to that stressful event (Walker *et al.*, 1989). A person gains a sense of control if they believe that they can bring some influence to bear on an aversive situation. This sense of control helps the person to cope with a stressful event. A number of authors have explored the link between sense of control and the pain experience. Bates *et al.* (1993) found that numerous patients with chronic pain reported a loss of sense of control as a result of their pain experience. In the Bates study of ethnocultural influences on variation in chronic pain perception they demonstrated that locus of control (LOC) style, along with ethnocultural affiliation were the best predictors of differences in pain intensity. People with an external LOC style experienced more intense pain than those with an internal LOC style. Many of the subjects reported that their pre-pain sense of control over life circumstances had been altered by their pain experience. Some patients managed to regain a sense of control over life circumstances despite the fact that they still were experiencing pain. The authors could not explain why this occurred but suggest that this is an important area for further study. Walker *et al.* (1990) have also demonstrated that external locus of control is a predictor of poorer levels of pain control. Pain intensity was associated with perceived control over pain. This has also been shown in a study of female patients undergoing surgery (Johnson *et al.*, 1989). Patients with external LOC experienced higher pain scores and also less satisfaction with their patient controlled analgesia (PCA).

There is evidence that feelings of helplessness are important predictors of higher levels of pain in patients with phantom limb pain (Hill *et al.*, 1995). It could be argued that feelings of helplessness are closely associated with a sense of poor control – those who feel helpless are unlikely to feel any mastery over a situation.

Lack of knowledge can influence a person's belief about whether they can control a situation (Walker *et al.*, 1989). A number of nursing research studies have shown that increasing patients' levels of knowledge through the provision of pre-operative information helped to give them a sense of control over a novel and extremely stressful situation (Hayward, 1975; Davis, 1984). This in turn resulted in a reduction in pain perception and analgesic consumption.

Previous experience with pain can also influence a person's sense of control over a situation. A positive experience with a previous painful situation will foster a sense of confidence and mastery over the situation. Conversely, if people have experienced unrelieved pain as a consequence of a procedure such as surgery, or an event such as childbirth, they may be apprehensive about their ability to control pain when confronted with similar situations in the future (Scott, 1994). This is why it is prudent to ensure that the first time a patient encounters any potentially painful procedure or event, that efforts are made to make it as painfree as possible.

Emotional state

A person's emotional state can be both a cause and a consequence of pain. A large number of studies have addressed this important issue, although there is no clear consensus on the nature of the relationship between different emotions and different types of pain. For example, Wade *et al.* (1990) found that anger and frustration, as opposed to anxiety, were important factors in the perception of chronic pain, whereas in a study of patients with chronic pain syndromes Gaskin *et al.* (1992) demonstrated that anxiety and anger contributed significantly to the degree of unpleasantness associated with the pain experience. These authors also found that chronic pain adversely affects mood states, as opposed to mood states predisposing to the development of chronic pain. By contrast, Bergbom Engberg *et al.* (1995) found that patients who experienced psychosocial stress, such as a relative's or spouse's illness or an extended period of feeling unhappy or depressed, at the time of onset of herpes zoster reported more severe pain than other patients.

Pain does not always adversely affect mood; other factors such as work and marital status can place chronic pain patients at greater risk of becoming depressed (Averil *et al.*, 1996). A study by Spiegel and Bloom (1983a) has shown that mood disturbance was a strong predictor of pain in women with metastatic breast cancer; however, these authors were unable to say whether the pain increased anxiety and depression or whether anxiety and depression caused the pain.

Anxiety is thought to have an important effect on postoperative pain perception. There are many reasons for people awaiting surgery to feel anxious. The mere fact of being hospitalised may provoke feelings of anxiety. Such anxiety is often compounded by fears of the possible outcome of impending surgery, in particular post-operative pain. Copp (1990) describes many of the anticipatory fears patients have about potentially painful procedures. She suggests that one of the most important fears is fear of the unknown and uses the following quote from Evely (1967) to illustrate this point:

'What is unbearable is not to suffer but to be afraid of suffering. To endure a precise pain, a definite loss, a hunger for something one knows – this is possible to bear. One can live with this pain. But in fear there is all the suffering of the world: to dread suffering is to suffer an infinite pain since one supposes it unbearable...'

This highlights the importance of allieviating fears through the provision of information and by dispelling misconceptions. Although a number of studies have demonstrated a positive relationship between anxiety and pain, other researchers have shown that anxiety may not necessarily increase pain in all situations (Al Absi & Rokke, 1991). These authors found that under experimental conditions, subjects who were anxious about an event which was irrelevant to the source of the pain reported less pain than those who were anxious about an event relevant to the source of their pain. Great caution should be exercised in extrapolating these findings to the clinical setting; nevertheless, it seems clear that the relationship between anxiety and pain perception is not unidirectional, and further study is required to elucidate the relationship.

Despite these ambiguous findings regarding the relationship between emotions and pain perception, it is important to draw some conclusions. There is adequate evidence to support the statement that patients with increased emotional distress, regardless of the cause, will report more pain. In clinical practice, however, it is prudent to identify which negative emotion is contributing to the patient's emotional distress and then to employ treatment approaches which are specific for that emotion (Gaskin *et al.*, 1992). If patients are anxious about a particular procedure, rather than making an attempt to reduce procedure-related anxiety, it may prove more fruitful to employ an alternative approach which aims at redirecting the focus of the patients' concerns (Al Absi & Rokke, 1991).

Gender

The degree to which a person's gender influences pain perception is by no means clear. A number of studies have shown that women both perceive and express more pain than men (Crook *et al.*, 1984; Feine *et al.*, 1991), whereas, other studies have demonstrated no differences between the sexes (Brattberg *et al.*, 1989; Bush *et al.*, 1993). Lautenbacher and Rollman (1993) demonstrated no difference between the sexes when heat or cold were applied, yet found that women had a significantly lower pain threshold to electrical stimuli. The degree to which these findings are relevant to clinical practice is questionable, since many of the studies have focused on experimentally-induced pain which employs a cutaneous stimulus. In clinical practice, it is more likely that patients will be suffering from deep somatic or visceral pain.

Studies suggest that women are more aware of health problems, will report symptoms more readily and be more willing to accept help than men (Bush *et al.*, 1993). Men tend to be less willing to report pain, particularly to females (Levine & De Simone, 1991). This may be because men want to impress women by being 'macho' or stoic in the face of pain. Although these studies were carried out in an experimental setting, these findings have implications for clinical practice. A male patient may find it difficult to admit pain to a female nurse, especially if he comes from a culture where the male macho role is highly valued.

4.5 Pain expression

There are a wide variety of physiological and behavioural manifestations of pain. Physiological manifestations of pain include a number of responses such as raised pulse and blood pressure, whereas behavioural manifestations are related to what people do or say in response to their pain (Meinhart & McCaffery, 1983).

Physiological manifestations of pain

A sequence of physiological reactions is thought to occur when a patient experiences pain (Table 4.1). These reactions are influenced by the person's normal response style and the intensity of the pain (Meinhart & McCaffery, 1983).

Table 4.1 Physiological responses to pain.

- Activation
- Rebound
- Adaptation
- Stress reaction

Activation occurs when a patient experiences an intense pain sensation of sudden onset. This reaction is the classical 'fight or flight' response of the body which results from activation of the sympathetic nervous system and is characterised by the presence of a number of physiological signs (Table 4.2). This response is sustained normally for a short period of time.

Table 4.2 Physiological responses during activation.

- Tachycardia
- Hypertension
- Cold perspiration
- Pallor
- Nausea
- Dilated pupils
- Piloerection
- Increase in muscle tension
- Reduced gastric secretion
- Decreased blood flow to viscera and skin

The body cannot sustain increased sympathetic function over a prolonged period of time and therefore some degree of adaptation usually occurs. This involves a decrease in sympathetic activity which results in less visible increases in blood pressure and pulse. If the pain sensation does not disappear, a general stress reaction will occur. This is characterised by increased adrenocortical activity which results in the production of higher concentrations of steroid hormones (Cox, 1978).

The increased production of steroid hormones is thought to fuel the activity of coping. Unfortunately, high concentrations of steroid hormones are not without negative effects which include impaired inflammatory response, interference with the manufacture of protein and raised blood sugar levels. During this time the patient's physiological response to pain will be minimal, although the intensity of that pain may remain unchanged. Thus, in the long term, physiological signs are poor indicators of pain.

Behavioural manifestations of pain

When people experience pain, they normally manifest a range of different behaviours including verbalisation, vocalisation, body movement and facial expression. It should not be assumed that overt behaviours are direct expressions of the intensity or quality of the pain experience (Sutters & Miaskowski, 1992). Pain is not always 'written all over a person's face'.

If we are to accept the principle that 'pain is what the patient says hurts', then verbalisation is the most important way for a person to communicate that they are in pain. However, some people, such as those who are cognitively impaired or those who do not speak the language of those around them, are unable to verbalise that they are in pain and they have to resort to vocalisations as a means of communication.

According to Meinhart and McCaffery (1983) vocalisations are all the sounds a patient may emit that are not language (Table 4.3). Vocalisations are used to great effect to communicate pain intensity, although they are probably used to a much lesser degree by those with chronic pain.

Table 4.3 Pain behaviours: vocalisations.

- Crying
- Moaning
- Groaning
- Gasping
- Whimpering
- Whining
- Screaming
- Sobbing

Patients use a range of body movements as a means of both expressing and controlling pain (Table 4.4). Some body movements are extremely effective at reducing pain intensity and in preventing pain returning, thereby ensuring maximum comfort. It is important to differentiate between pain expression behaviours and pain control behaviours; otherwise the significance of a particular body movement may be misinterpreted (Wilkie *et al.*, 1989).

Table 4.4 Pain behaviours: body movements.

- Limping
- Rubbing the affected part
- Applying pressure to the affected body area
- Immobilisation
- Protective movement
- Inaccurate body movement
- Restlessness
- Supporting the painful body part

Many researchers have demonstrated that adults and children from a Western culture who are experiencing acute pain manifest a typical facial expression (Table 4.5) (LeResche, 1982; LeResche & Dworkin, 1984; Prkachin, 1992). There is no evidence to demonstrate that a typical facial expression exists for those in chronic pain, those who are confused and those from different cultures (LeResche & Dworkin, 1984; Closs, 1994).

Table 4.5 Pain behaviours: facial expressions.

- Brow lowering
- Clenched teeth
- Horizontally stretched open mouth
- Closed eyes
- Orbit tightening

4.6 Factors which influence the person's expression of pain

Adaptation

As mentioned previously, the body will not sustain a physiological response to pain in the long term. Therefore, if pain is persistant, it is likely that the pronounced physiological signs which accompany acute pain will revert to normal. Moreover, many patients will learn to modify their behavioural responses to pain. They do this for a number of reasons. It may be that patients are so fatigued from their pain experience that they do not have enough energy to express pain (McCaffrey, 1980; McCaffrey & Beebe, 1994). It is also possible that patients soon learn that certain pain expressions, which are acceptable when in acute pain, become unacceptable when pain persists in the long term (Eland, 1978). To survive patients must modify their normal pain expressions. This process takes hard work and long periods of time.

Some patients adapt their behaviours because they have found over time that certain behaviours such as sleeping, watching television, reading or talking to friends help to make their pain bearable (Wilkie *et al.*, 1989). They use these behaviours to take their mind off their pain, often with great effect. Adaptation is not always associated with such beneficial behaviours. Some people in chronic pain manifest a range of behaviours similar to those seen in depression (Twycross, 1994). Regardless of which of the above mentioned behaviours a person manifests, healthcare professionals need to be careful not to misinterpret them as a sign that the patient is not in pain.

Difficulties with verbalising pain

Some patients are unable to verbalise pain because of language barriers, a physical disability which impairs speech or cognitive impairment. However, even those who can communicate verbally or who are cognitively sound, may experience some difficulty when verbalising their pain. It is often difficult to find a word or words which describe adequately the nature of some pains. As Scarry (1985) points out, 'Physical pain does not simply resist language but actively destroys it.' Patients may not even use the word 'pain' to describe a pain experience (Francke & Theeuwen, 1994). They often use other terms such as 'discomfort', 'heaviness', 'unpleasant feeling', 'soreness', 'pressure' to describe pain, particularly that which is less intense or chronic in nature. Providing patients with a list of pain descriptors may give them the vocabulary they need to describe their pain.

Beliefs and attitudes

Patients may be reluctant to express pain because of a variety of different beliefs and attitudes they hold about pain and its treatments. Yates *et al.* (1995) found that patients were reluctant to discuss their pain with a number of different people. For example, they were reluctant to discuss pain with their significant others for fear of worrying them. Patients hid their pain from staff because they believed that staff were too busy to help and they didn't want to cause any bother. The attitude of staff also influenced the degree to which patients are willing to express pain. If staff do not appear to be interested in listening to patients' complaints of pain, it is unlikely that patients will bother expressing pain.

If patients hold very fatalistic beliefs about the inevitability of their pain and the possibility of controlling it, they may stop complaining of pain because they feel 'why bother, I just have to put up with it, nothing can be done about it anyway' (Francke & Theeuwen, 1994; Ward & Gatwood, 1994; Yates *et al.*, 1995). Patients hold a wide variety of other misconceptions, beliefs and fears about pain and its treatment. Clearly, these have a significant impact on a patient's willingness to express pain to healthcare professionals. Further discussion on this issue can be found in Chapter 5.

Secondary gains

If a person gains any practical, financial or emotional advantage from their pain, they may express it more frequently. Such advantages are referred to as secondary gains, a term which should not be confused with malingering, since the patient is not lying about the presence of pain (McCaffrey & Beebe, 1994). In this situation pain is often used by patients as a way of 'opting out' of dealing with problems or of avoiding undesirable situations and activities. It may also be used as a means of eliciting social support or of controlling situations (Walker *et al.*, 1989; Snelling, 1994). A vicious circle can develop when this behaviour is positively reinforced by family members (Snelling, 1994).

In the long term secondary gain can result in social isolation, lack of occupation, strain in family relationships, marital conflicts and physical disability; therefore, if patients are using pain in a dysfunctional manner, efforts should be made to facilitate them to develop more positive coping strategies. Moreover, family members should be helped to develop ways of responding more effectively to their relatives' behaviour.

Personality

Personality can affect how a person expresses pain. Introverts are often reluctant to complain of pain, whereas extroverts are more likely to complain of pain (Bond & Pearson, 1969) and therefore to receive more medication. This may be because extroverts tolerate pain less well. The degree to which one can generalise the effect of personality on the expression of different types of pain is unclear (Heath & Thomas, 1993). Nevertheless, it seems wise to assess the patient's normal reaction to pain, illness and stress so that assumptions are not made about the pain being experienced.

Culture

In every culture pain acquires a specific social significance, and therefore a knowledge of each culture's attitude towards pain is important in understanding individual reactions (Zborowski, 1979). Zborowski (1979) considers three different types of pain: self-inflicted, others-inflicted and spontaneous. He defines self-inflicted pain as deliberately and voluntarily self-inflicted and usually having a culturally defined purpose. An example of this would be drawing blood with a knife as part of an initiation rite. Others-inflicted pain is pain inflicted by others upon the individual whilst undertaking culturally accepted activities, such as sport and fighting. Finally, he defines spontaneous pain as that which results from disease or injury.

Different cultures may hold differing attitudes towards each type of pain. Two such attitudes include pain acceptance and pain expectancy. Pain acceptance is characterised by a willingness to experience pain, whereas pain expectancy is the anticipation of pain in a particular situation such as childbirth. Some cultures will expect pain but will not accept it. For example, in the United States, labour pain is expected but not accepted, whereas in other cultures labour pain is both expected and accepted. In the former situation various means are employed to relieve pain and in the latter, little is done to alleviate it. Thus, when exploring the impact of culture on pain expression, consideration needs to be given to the type of pain involved and that culture's expectancy and acceptance of the pain. Pain expression is often dictated by a culture's attitude towards pain *per se* or the type of pain being experienced. Other social norms of pain behaviour based on age, sex and social position are also important. For example, it has been found that a stoic reaction to pain is idealised by the Bariba of Benin tribe whose members are expected to demonstrate a non-expressive response to pain across a number of life situations (Sargent, 1984). In this situation the behaviour in response to pain was learned; people expressed less pain even though they may not have felt less pain.

A number of studies have examined the impact of culture on pain expression, although this literature is limited by the fact that it is mostly North American in origin. Zola (1975) compared Irish and Italians and found that the Irish were more likely to deny that pain was a feature of their illness. When asked directly about their pain the Irish hedged their replies with qualifications (e.g. 'it was more of a throbbing than a pain … not really pain'). The Italians tended to report more pain and information about the impact of the pain on their life in general. Zola suggested that these differences may exist because in Irish culture denial and restraint are the *modus operandi* for handling troubles, whereas Italians, particularly those from the South, deal with theirs by generalisation and drama-tisation.

Zborowski (1979) has also explored the role of cultural components in the pain experience. He studied the way men of Jewish, Italian, and 'Old American' (northern European) descent reacted to pain and their attitudes towards pain. He found that Italians and Jews tended to express their pain more freely and were not ashamed by this expression. However, the Jewish and Italian subjects held quite different attitudes towards their pain; and even though they expressed pain in a similar way, their expressions served different purposes. By contrast, Old Americans were much more stoical and unemotional when expressing pain. Pain was minimised and there was a tendency to avoid complaining since complaining 'wouldn't help anyone' and the patient wanted to avoid being a 'nuisance'.

In a study of inter-ethnic differences in pain perception Greenwald (1991) found a significant variation in how people from different ethnic groups expressed pain in emotional terms. People of English, German and Scandinavian (Old American) origin had low scores on the McGill Pain Questionnaire affective subscale. This supports Zborowski's and Zola's earlier work. Interestingly, Greenwald (1991) found no inter-ethnic difference in pain perception.

Bates and her colleagues (1993) also found significant inter-ethnic differences in emotional responses to chronic pain. They found that Hispanics believed emotional expressions of pain were an appropriate response to pain, whereas Old Americans and Poles felt that non-expression was the ideal response. These authors also found significant intra-ethnic group differences in pain response and concluded, therefore, that it is inappropriate to stereotype patients from certain ethnic groups. Nonetheless, they do highlight the importance of acknowledging cultural differences in pain expression – otherwise the clinician runs the risk of making a poor clinical decision.

Despite its limitations, there is a body of evidence which indicates that people from different cultures express pain differently. However, there is a danger of stereotyping people according to their ethnic group, as there is significant variation in pain expression within ethnic groups. Garro (1990) suggests that older people, particularly women, identify more closely with their cultural traditions. This should be borne in mind when assessing people in pain.

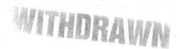

Summary of Chapter 4

- Pain is a fundamental and inevitable form of human suffering, the experience of which is unique to each individual.
- Pain is not merely a bodily experience; it is a phenomenon which is modulated by physical, psychological, social, cultural and spiritual factors.
- The concept of pain threshold incorporates a number of phenomena including the lowest limit at which a sensation is perceptible or feels painful and the highest limit at which a sensation is bearable or the person asks for it to be withdrawn.
- People can be encouraged to tolerate a painful sensation, a situation which can be exploited to the patient's benefit in clinical practice.
- Pain can have a range of different meanings for people – some cancer patients equate increasing levels of pain with disease progression and impending death, whereas pain from an injury is often viewed as a nuisance which will go away eventually.
- People who view their pain in a negative way can often find it difficult to accept. In contrast, people who view their pain in a more positive light can often cope more effectively with their pain.
- Cultural background can influence both pain expression and the meaning that patients attribute to a pain experience.
- Religious beliefs, feelings of loss, or emotional state can cause some people to view pain positively, others to view it in a negative way.
- Gender may influence pain perception although it is more likely to influence pain expression.
- A person will not sustain a physiological response to pain in the long term. Thus the pronounced physiological signs which accompany acute pain are not seen in patients with chronic pain.
- Patients can have difficulties in verbalising pain because of language barriers, a speech impairment, cognitive impairment, or they may be reluctant to express pain because of cultural beliefs.
- If a person gains any practical, financial or emotional advantage from their pain, they may express it more frequently.
- There is a danger of stereotyping patients according to culture, personality or gender, as there is significant variation in pain expression within these groups.

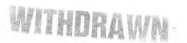
WITHDRAWN

Chapter 5

Barriers to Effective Pain Management

In their book *Defeating Pain: The War Against a Silent Epidemic*, Wall and Jones (1991) provide a summary of an ombudsman's report about an incident which occurred in March 1988 in a National Health Service hospital. An 85-year-old woman who had been admitted to a London teaching hospital with a fractured thigh was in such severe pain one night, that she cried out for help. The response from her nurse was to move the woman to a dark room with no bell or light switch. According to the woman's son, 'She lay there begging for help in the darkness, the pain becoming worse in her leg... She was left there, she thinks, for about 4 to 6 hours'. Wall and Jones posed the question 'How could such a shocking incident have occurred?' An immediate answer might be that the nurse was not prepared to do anything about the elderly lady's pain. But could it be that the nurse just felt powerless to do anything about the pain?

How often do we allow patients to experience unnecessary suffering? Studies suggest that we do so with unacceptable frequency (Marks & Sacher, 1973; Cohen, 1980; Donovan *et al.*, 1987; Seers, 1987; Alleyne & Thomas, 1994). This is despite the fact that we have both the means and the knowledge to ameliorate pain effectively. A cursory inspection of the literature or evidence from everyday clinical practice provide numerous examples of the subtle and complicated barriers that can contribute to poor treatment of pain. These barriers are summarised in Table 5.1 and include poor training of healthcare professionals, myths and misconceptions about pain and the use of opioids, and problems with the healthcare system. This chapter explores these barriers in greater depth and identifies ways in which they can be overcome.

5.1 Factors related to healthcare professionals

Lack of knowledge

There is ample evidence to demonstrate that both nurses and doctors have poor knowledge about pain and its management (Cohen, 1980; McCaffrey *et al.*, 1990; Diekmann & Wassem, 1991; Vortherms *et al.*, 1992; Fothergill-Bourbonnais & Wilson-Barnett, 1992; Jose Closs, 1996). It is

Table 5.1   Common reasons for unrelieved pain.

Fault with healthcare professionals
- Poor knowledge about the nature of pain and its management
- Poor pain assessment
  - inadequate collection of data
  - poor recognition of the multi-dimensional nature of pain
  - poor timing of assessment
  - poor interpretation of data
  - underutilisation of pain measurement tools
  - poor documentation
- Poor utilisation of pain management skills
- Myths and misconceptions about opioids
  - fear of addiction and respiratory depression
  - fear of tolerance
  - misconceptions about the placebo response
  - ageism

Fault with patients and family members
- Reluctance to report pain
  - desire to be a 'good' patient
  - fear of addiction with opioids
  - fatalistic attitudes about pain management
  - fear that pain means that disease is progressing
  - belief that pain builds character
  - view pain as having moral value
- Non-compliance with treatment
  - lack of understanding
  - desire to maintain some control of the situation
  - belief that analgesic agents should only be taken if absolutely necessary
  - belief that strong pain medication should be saved until the pain gets really bad

Fault with healthcare system
- Barriers to opioid availability
  - bureaucratic regulations about prescribing opioids
  - unwillingness of pharmacies to stock opioids
- Breakdowns in continuity of care
  - poor system of organising nursing work
  - poor co-ordination of care between different healthcare settings
  - low priority given to pain management
  - lack of accountability for pain management

also clear that contemporary nursing and medical education programmes do not equip healthcare professionals with sufficient knowledge about:

- the nature and causes of pain;
- the difference between acute and chronic pain;
- the effects of different factors on pain perception and expression;

- methods of pain assessment;
- the pharmacology of analgesics;
- the principles of pain management.

Not suprisingly, this situation results in many professionals feeling ill-prepared to care for patients in pain (Fothergill-Bourbonnais & Wilson-Barnett, 1992; Alleyne & Thomas, 1994). More worrying, however, is that insufficient knowledge compromises a nurse's ability to make optimal clinical decisions and fosters an environment where ritualistic practices thrive (Walsh & Ford, 1989). Examples of poor decision making and ritualistic practices commonly encountered include:

- underestimation of the severity of the patient's pain;
- overestimation of the effectiveness of interventions;
- establishing inappropriate treatment goals;
- administering a lower dose of analgesic at longer intervals than pre-scribed;
- reluctance to administer parenteral analgesics;
- withholding analgesics prescribed on a fixed time-interval basis when the patient is not in pain;
- administering the lowest dose of analgesic possible as opposed to the dose required to control the pain (Cohen, 1980; White, 1985; Dono-van *et al.*, 1987; Seers, 1987; Carr, 1990; Harrison, 1991).

Lack of knowledge about pain and its management can be exacerbated by the fact that nurses do not commonly utilise research findings in their everyday clinical practice (Dufault *et al.*, 1995). One reason proposed for this is that nurses do not know how to interpret research findings and do not have a very positive attitude towards research. Thus, not only is it necessary to improve nurses' knowledge about pain and its management, it is also important to improve their competency in interpreting research and utilising relevant findings.

Doctors are also capable of making poor clinical decisions due to lack of knowledge, the most common being a failure to prescribe appropriate therapeutic interventions and poor monitoring of the patient's response to treatment. The dose of opioid prescribed for patients is sometimes well below therapeutic levels (Marks & Sacher, 1973; Weis *et al.*, 1983; Donovan *et al.*, 1987; Donovan, 1989). This situation can prove very frustrating for nurses, since doctors control the prescription of analgesics. Alleyne and Thomas (1994) provide a distressing account of a nurse attempting to persuade the doctor that a patient really had pain and required more analgesia. Such scenarios are probably repeated across many healthcare settings and highlight the lack of power nurses sometimes experience in clinical decision making.

It is clear that these poor practices arise for a number of inter-related reasons. However lack of knowledge would appear to be a central issue, and addressing this barrier must be a priority in tackling the problem of poor pain management.

Poor pain assessment

Inadequate collection of data

A good assessment is the cornerstone of effective symptom control, yet current pain assessment practices leave much to be desired. Nurses' perceptions of patients' pain are often quite different from those of their patients in that they have a tendency to overestimate the levels of least pain, underestimate the levels of worst pain and overestimate the effectiveness of interventions (Seers, 1987; Camp, 1988; Choiniere *et al.*, 1990; Grossman *et al.*, 1991; O'Connor, 1995a; O'Connor 1995b). What appears to be happening is that nurses make inferences about a patient's pain on the basis of what they observe. This is not problematic if the nurse confirms the validity of these inferences with the patient, but all too often this is not done. Some nurses do not even ask the patient 'Are you in pain?', nor do they confirm the intensity of the pain (Donovan, *et al.*, 1987). Even if nurses do ask patients if they are in pain, they may not get a clear and unambiguous response.

This may be because the question is worded ambiguously, is not sufficiently searching, or it may be that patients do not always use the word 'pain' unless their pain is very severe (Francke and Theeuwen, 1994). Indeed, it has been shown that a general question does not adequately assess pain (Cohen, 1980). Take for example, a patient who does not experience pain when lying still, yet experienced pain on movement; the patient would answer 'no' to the question about being in pain when lying still, and if the nurse did not pursue the question any further, the pain on movement would be completely missed (Carr, 1990).

Assessment of pain is complicated further because nurses often assume that patients will complain of pain, whereas patients expect the nurse to enquire about their pain (Seers, 1987; Franke & Theeuwen, 1994). There is evidence that some patients do not spontaneously report their pain to other people (Wilkie *et al.*, 1995). In addition, there is no guarantee that even if patients do spontaneously complain of pain that they will provide clinically relevant information (Harrison, 1991). This is because most patients lack specialist knowledge and therefore, do not know what information about their pain would help healthcare professionals make more accurate clinical decisions (Wilkie *et al.*, 1995). Thus, even if the nurse asks the question 'How is your pain?', the patient may not be able to provide significant information without some guidance. Unfortunately, even when patients are guided to report certain information about their pain, some may not be able to convey the reality of their experience because they are unable to find words which adequately describe it (Scarry, 1985).

Nurses often experience difficulties when communicating with patients, especially those who are terminally ill. These difficulties can lead to the use of blocking tactics, which prevent patients from sharing information about their problems and which will in turn compromise the assessment process. The results from one study which explored how nurses communicate with cancer patients clearly demonstrated that nurses only carry out very superficial physical assessments. They were able to identify distressing symptoms, yet made little attempt to elicit the intensity of each symptom or the degree to which it affected the patient (Wilkinson, 1991). Thus, if nurses experience difficulty or lack skills in communicating with patients, it is possible that any pain assessment they undertake will be superficial and interventions will be planned on the basis of incomplete information.

Poor recognition of the multi-dimensional nature of pain

The multi-dimensional nature of pain is often poorly recognised by professionals. As a result, only the physical cause of the pain is focused on, and the capacity of emotional, spiritual and social factors to influence a person's experience of pain is not acknowledged. This lack of understanding may be manifested in a number of erroneous beliefs – for instance, that the same tissue damage should produce the same pain in different people (Harrison, 1991); or the belief that if a physical cause for pain cannot be found, the pain is 'all in the head'; or that the patient is lying (Cassel, 1982; McCaffrey, 1980).

Clearly, if efforts are focused on searching for a physical cause for pain or on controlling physical pain, without consideration of the other factors, it is highly unlikely that optimal pain control will be achieved (O'Brien, 1993). As Saunders (1988) points out, 'We have to learn to listen in a way that will help the suffering person find the route to the real trouble, and the way to face and handle it.' This is of particular importance in patients with chronic pain.

Poor timing of assessment

Assessment of pain can be compromised by using routine drug rounds as the time for pain assessment. It is quite obvious that an assessment carried out by a nurse standing at a drug trolley in the middle of a ward will be much more superficial than if the nurse sat down quietly by the patient's side (Carr, 1990). An additional difficulty associated with carrying out a pain assessment during the drug round may be that some patients feel compelled to take analgesics at this time because they know the trolley will not be back for another four hours (Sofaer,1992). Such fixed routines of pain assessment and analgesic administration deny individual differences between patients (Hayward, 1975). More worrying is the fact that they may result in some nurses disbelieving their patients if they complain of pain at other times (Wakefield, 1995) or in some patients not requesting analgesics for fear of bothering the nurses (Sofaer, 1992).

Poor interpretation of data

Incorrect interpretation of non-verbal cues can contribute greatly to poor assessments. Nurses often assume that if patients look comfortable or are sleeping, then they must be pain free. Furthermore, they often expect patients in pain to manifest certain behaviours and physiological signs. Some pain control behaviours, such as watching television or talking to friends, are easily misinterpreted as an indication that the patient is not in pain (Wilkie *et al.*, 1989). Patients exhibiting more expressive pain behaviours such as crying, moaning and facial expressions of suffering can be perceived by nurses as being more distressed than stoical patients (Von Baeyer *et al.*, 1984).

It seems then that in the absence of certain physiological signs and expected pain behaviours, nurses may doubt that the patient's pain is in any way severe. Yet overt behaviours and signs of autonomic stimulation are not always good indicators of pain intensity or quality (Sutters & Miaskowski, 1992). This is particularly so with chronic pain since the body is incapable of sustaining increased autonomic function over a prolonged period of time, and some degree of adaptation normally occurs. Moreover, most patients with severe pain will manage to achieve some degree of uninterrupted sleep (Donovan *et al.*, 1987).

As discussed in Chapter 4, a patient's cultural background can also have a profound influence on pain expression (Garro, 1990; Bates *et al.*, 1993). Clearly, it is important to be aware of how culture can influence pain expression; however, it is also important to remember that there will be significant variation in pain expression within cultural groups. There is a similar risk of error if people are stereotyped according to their culture, or indeed other factors such as age, gender or socio-economic status. Nurses should take into account that each patient will have a unique response to pain which will be influenced by many factors. It is very easy to under-estimate or overestimate a person's pain if the assessment is based on observation alone, and such errors will only be prevented by placing greater emphasis on what patients have to say about their pain.

Nurses' own cultural background may also influence the degreee to which they infer suffering in their patients. There is evidence that nurses from various backgrounds differ in their inferences of both physical pain and psychological distress (Davitz & Davitz, 1985). For example, nurses from Nepal and Taiwan have been shown to rate psychological distress very low, yet pain quite high. Conversely, Puerto Rican nurses rate psychological distress very highly, but give a quite low rate to pain, and English nurses give both physical pain and psychological distress very low ratings. These findings may reflect the norms in relation to pain expression in the respective nurse's culture. For instance, in Puerto Rico it is normal to be very expressive when in pain, but this does not necessarily mean that a person is extremely distressed. In Chinese culture attaining a level of 'inner peace' is rewarded, and in British culture maintaining a 'stiff upper lip' is valued.

The implications of this study are important. Nurses may not assess pain or suffering very well in patients from a cultural background which is different from their own. Nurses who come from a culture where dramatic expressions of pain are abnormal may have difficulty accepting that someone is in pain and may consider patients to be overly demanding and time consuming. As a result patients may feel rejected and nurses stressed and irritated. Similarly if patients' culturally determined pain expressions do not reveal the depths of their suffering and they are being cared for by nurses from a culture where dramatic expressions of pain are the norm, there is a risk that the patients' pain will be overlooked. Clearly, nurses need to recognise the degree to which their own cultural biases influence their assessment of pain (Davitz & Davitz, 1985).

Level of experience may influence nurses inference of pain. Nurses with limited clinical experience have been shown to infer a higher degree of physical suffering than more experienced nurses (Mason, 1981). Other studies have also shown that experienced nurses are more likely to understate their patients' pain (Dudley & Holm, 1984; Lander, 1990; Choiniere *et al.*, 1990). There are a number of reasons put forward as explanations for this phenomenon. Some suggest that nurses may become desensitised after repeated exposure to patients' physical suffering, others that nurses play down their patients' pain in order to protect themselves from becoming emotionally drained as a result of witnessing excessive amounts of suffering (Harrison, 1991).

It is important to acknowledge the difficulty of remaining with someone in pain, particularly when the pain is one for which we feel we can do nothing. Some pains are extremely difficult to ameliorate, and others will never go away, which can be extremely frustrating for the healthcare team who may feel a deep sense of failure. This in itself may cause the team to 'turn their back' on the patient. Saunders (1988) recommends that in these situations we should 'persevere with the practical'. This may be all we have to offer some patients, but in persevering we may just help the patient come to terms with their new reality and continue to live their lives in a way that is acceptable to them. Sometimes there are no easy answers.

Under-utilisation of pain measurement tools

One means of overcoming the problem of inadequate collection and interpretation of data is through the use of pain measurement tools. Measurement tools provide objective measures of different dimensions of the pain experience (see discussion in Chapter 6), but more importantly, they facilitate patients in communicating their pain experience and providing evidence of that experience which is very difficult for healthcare professionals to ignore. Unfortunately, across a range of clinical settings, there is much evidence to show that pain assessment tools are rarely used in everyday practice (Couveur, 1990; Walker *et al.*, 1990; Hollingsworth, 1995). It seems clear then that significant efforts are required to encourage healthcare professionals to use measurement tools as a fundamental component of the pain assessment process.

Poor documentation

Information about patients' pain is often recorded inaccurately, incompletely and inconsistently. Nurses have problems with recording information regarding the duration, intensity and quality of pain (O'Connor, 1995a; 1995b), the progress of the patient's pain (Donovan *et al.*, 1987), and the patient's perception of their pain (Camp, 1988). If clinically relevant pieces of information are not documented and the nurse who has collected that information is unavailable, at best, the patient will be inconvenienced by being asked the same set of questions again, at worst, incorrect clinical decisions will be made about the patient's pain.

Poor documentation of pain may be a reflection of poor documentation in nursing *per se*, as there is ample evidence available to demonstrate that nurses are not good at documenting patient care (de la Cuesta, 1983; Suhayda & Kim, 1984; Davis *et al.*, 1994). Unfortunately, there are many factors associated with poor documentation in nursing, which means that bringing about improvements in nurses' documentary practices may be an uphill struggle. This difficulty was clearly demonstrated by Camp-Sorrell and O'Sullivan (1991) who found that a short continuing education programme on pain assessment and the documentation of that assessment did not improve documentary practices to any significant degree. Nurses did not think that pain was sufficiently important to merit complete assessment and documentation.

Improving pain assessment

Clearly continuing education has an important role in facilitating nurses to develop better pain assessment skills. Careful planning needs to go into the development of such programmes because studies have shown that some of the approaches adopted in the past are not very successful. For instance, a training programme which aimed at helping nurses to develop better assessment skills only had a limited impact on their ability to identify their patients' concerns (Heaven & Maguire, 1996). This may be because simple skills training is insufficient to change clinical behaviour, and other factors such as challenging nurses' attitudes and beliefs about their own communication skills should also be addressed in training programmes.

Continuing education programmes may prove to be more beneficial if they are aimed at not only increasing knowledge about pain and its management but also at helping nurses to become more sensitive to their patients' pain (McCaffrey & Ferrell, 1997). This suggestions is based on evidence that decision making about pain and its management is influenced by whether the nurse assumes a personal or professional role. It has been shown that when nurses were presented with a vignette of a patient who reports that he is in pain, those nurses who assumed a 'sibling' role were more sensitive to the patient's pain and his need for pain relief (McCaffrey & Ferrell, 1997).

Poor utilisation of pain management skills

Nurses may be knowledgeable about the beneficial effect of some interventions, yet this is not a guarantee that they will employ such interventions with their own patients. For example, Dalton (1989) demonstrated that nurses are aware of the role that complementary therapies have in ameliorating pain; unfortunately they are not using them in their everyday clinical practice. There may be many reasons for this, including lack of time, lack of permission to use these therapies or the mere fact that nurses do not possess the skills to provide complementary therapies in a safe manner. As complementary therapies gain greater acceptance, it is probable that many of these problems will be addressed and that more nurses will attempt to further their skills in this area, particulary in the use of aromatherapy and massage (Closs, 1996).

Preoperative information giving provides another good example of where nurses do not always use beneficial interventions in practice. There is ample evidence to demonstrate that preoperative information giving helps to reduce postoperative pain (Hayward, 1975; Boore, 1978; Davis, 1984). However, nurses do not always become involved with preoperative information giving (Carr, 1990). This may be because they feel ill-prepared to undertake this role. On the other hand, it may be because nurses do not believe that they have a major role to play in information giving.

Myths and misconceptions

Ignorance about pain and its management has provided a fertile breeding ground for the development of some quite extraordinary myths and misconceptions (Table 5.2), which can contribute significantly to irrational clinical decision making. Cultural background and professional experience often reinforce these beliefs. For example, if most of the cancer patients you have cared for have experienced uncontrolled, excruciating

Table 5.2 Myths and misconceptions held by healthcare professionals about pain and its management.

- All pains have an identifiable physical cause.
- People with the same tissue damage should experience similar levels of pain.
- Patients not manifesting expected pain behaviours are not in pain.
- Patients who are sleeping are not in pain.
- Patients who are in pain will let the nurse know about it.
- Some pain (e.g. cancer pains) are inevitable and intractable.
- Opioids should be reserved until the pain is really bad.
- Non-pharmacological interventions are only effective for mild pain.
- Patients taking opioids on a prolonged basis become addicted.
- The use of opioids for pain is associated with clinically significant respiratory depression.
- Patients who come from areas where drug abuse is a common problem are more likely to become addicted.
- Pain relief following a placebo indicates that the patient is lying about their pain.
- Elderly patients experience less pain than younger people.
- Infants do not experience pain.

pain, you will possibly hold the fatalistic belief that cancer pain is inevitable and intractable.

Fear of addiction

Opioids are the most powerful analgesics available; yet their use is too often restricted because of unfounded fears and misconceptions. Indeed, fear of addiction or 'opiophobia' is one of the most frequently cited reasons for poor management of pain (McCaffrey, 1992). The incidence of addiction after use of opioid drugs for pain control is thought to be less than one percent (Porter & Jick, 1980); yet many healthcare professionals have exaggerated fears about the possibility of a patient becoming addicted (Marks & Sacher, 1973; Cohen, 1980; Fox, 1982; Weis *et al.*, 1983; McCaffrey *et al.*, 1990; Diekmann & Wassem, 1991). Opiophobia may be exaggerated further when patients are young or come from a culture where drug misuse is a common problem (Alleyne & Thomas, 1994). Fear of addiction can cause nurses to delay deliberately the provision of analgesics or to give less medication than ordered.

Opiophobia

The irrational and undocumented fear that appropriate use of opioid drugs causes addiction (Morgan, 1985).

It is paradoxical that patients with inadequately controlled pain may display behaviours which are similar to those seen in individuals who are psychologically dependent (addicted) on opioids. Patients may manifest behaviours such as 'clock watching', be overly concerned about the availability of analgesics or they may frequently request analgesics. This iatrogenic syndrome has been labelled as 'opioid pseudo-addiction' (Weissman & Haddox, 1989). Patients in pain who manifest drug seeking behaviours are sometimes perceived by healthcare professionals as 'becoming overly fond of their pain medication', a powerful euphemism for 'becoming addicted'. This in turn may compromise the care the patient receives and cause irrevocable damage to the relationship between the patient and healthcare professionals.

The problem of achieving effective control of pain is further compounded by the fact that patients and families share similar fears about addiction (Levin *et al.*, 1985; Weissman & Dahl, 1990). The myth of addiction has been fuelled by the war society is waging against drug misuse. Programmes such as the 'Just Say No' programme in the United States and films such as *Trainspotting* have sent out a strong message to the general public about the catastrophic impact of drugs on people's lives and that drugs such as heroin or morphine should be avoided at all costs. In the present antidrug culture it is not surprising that myths about addiction have arisen and that some patients, often with prompting from their relatives, refuse to take opioids. Clearly, a significant degree of public and professional education is necessary to overcome opiophobia. Perhaps the most important message to get over to the public and professionals alike is from the working party of the Royal College of Surgeons and Anaesthetists (1990):

> '...those that administer opioids are at greater risk of developing addiction than those who receive them'.

An important first step in public and professional education is the clarification of the term addiction, which means different things to different people. Technically the term means both physical and psychological dependence. However, many people interpret the term addiction as meaning psychological dependence alone – that is, the situation where the person obtains and uses drugs for their psychological effects, not for approved medical reasons. Such psychological dependence is often accompanied by physical dependence. People in pain who take opioids in the long term do develop physical dependence on these drugs, as do people who take corticosteriods in the long term. It is strange that we never use the term addiction to describe the physical dependence associated with corticosteriods, yet withdrawal symptoms, which are often life threatening, will accompany sudden cessation of these drugs (Wilkes *et al.*, 1994).

Patients who take opioids on a prolonged basis can also develop tolerance. The concept of tolerance should not be confused with that of dependence. Tolerance, which occurs with a number of different drugs, is where the body becomes 'used' to the effects of a drug following prolonged or frequent use and larger doses of a drug are necessary to maintain its original effect. It is important to note the difference between tolerance to the main pharmacological effect of a drug, which is the concept referred to above, and tolerance to the side effects of that drug. Tolerance will occur to many of the side effects of opioids; however, it will occur at a different rate for each side effect. For example, tolerance to euphoria develops quickly, but tolerance to gastro-intestinal effects is much slower. It should also be noted that patients may require an increased dose of a drug for reasons other than tolerance. For example, the most common reason for patients with advanced cancer to require more opioids is the fact that their disease is progressing, resulting in further tissue destruction.

Clearly, no matter how much opioid a patient in pain is receiving, it is totally inappropriate to label him or her as an addict. The connotations associated with the use of this term, even though it may be pharmacologically correct, can create an insurmountable barrier to effective pain management. A definition of addiction, tolerance and physical dependence is offered in Table 5.3. The definition of addiction may not be strictly technically correct, but may help clarify in people's minds that psychological dependence is not a problem when opioids are used for legitimate purposes.

Fear of tolerance

Fear of addiction is intimately linked with fear of tolerance. Some doctors are reluctant to prescribe opioids for patients with terminal illness, such as cancer, believing that if they initiate opioid therapy too soon there will be

Table 5.3   Definition of addiction, tolerance and physical dependence.

Addiction (psychological dependence)
An overwhelming and compulsive need to obtain and use drugs for their psychic effects, not for approved medical reasons (e.g. pain relief).

Tolerance
With prolonged or frequent use the body becomes 'used to' the effect of a drug and no longer responds to the same extent. A larger dose of drug is therefore required to maintain its original effect.

Physical dependence
A state that develops as the result of adaptation of the body to repeated drug use (tolerance). If the drug is stopped abruptly or an antagonist of that drug is administered, the body needs to re-adjust and withdrawal symptoms occur. The appearance of withdrawal symptoms is the only real evidence that dependence exists.

nothing stronger to prescribe 'when things get really bad'. They assume that tolerance to analgesia will develop and the opioids will be of no further benefit to the patient. This myth arises from a lack of knowledge of the normal dose range of opioids which can be employed in patients with advanced cancer.

A vicious circle can ensue where doctors fear prescribing opioids because according to their limited knowledge, they can only prescribe a small amount of opioid and tolerance will develop rapidly to this drug. They will then have to witness the patient's pain getting worse, which can leave them feeling totally impotent. Some key facts need to be conveyed to health professionals in order to eradicate this myth. It is true that some degree of tolerance to opioids will occur with prolonged use (see discussion below on Fear of Addiction); however, the reason most patients require an increase in their opioid dose is that their disease is progressing and this causes more pain (McCaffrey, 1992). Regardless of whether it is tolerance or disease progression which is causing increased pain, it is perfectly acceptable to administer very large doses of opioids to patients with advanced cancer, if this is what is required to control their pain.

Fear of respiratory depression

A misconception which also accompanies fear of addiction and tolerance is fear of respiratory depression. Respiratory depression as a result of opioid administration is an uncommon side effect which is reversible through the use of an opioid antagonist, such as naloxone. Moreover, since pain itself is a stimulus to respiration, respiratory depression will not feature as a problem until pain has been controlled. Despite these facts a great fear of respiratory depressions persists amongst healthcare professionals. An example of how this fear influences clinical practice was reported recently by Peate (1996) who questioned nurses about the factors which influenced their decisions regarding patient medication. One of the nurses replied that she withheld diamorphine from a terminally-ill patient because his breathing was laboured and that the last terminally-ill patient she had cared for with erratic breathing died ten minutes following administration of diamorphine.

Fear of respiratory depression also persists in postoperative and care-of-the-elderly settings. Many nurses believe that the administration of opioids post-operatively compromises patients' respiratory function (Cohen, 1980). They seem to overlook the fact that undermedication with opioids which results in increased pain is more likely to cause respiratory difficulties. Furthermore, a great many nurses believe that elderly patients who receive opioids for acute pain are at risk of developing clinically significant respiratory depression (Closs, 1996). However, there is little evidence to demonstrate that respiratory depression is a significant problem in elderly patients receiving opioids. Elderly patients often have Cheyne-Stokes breathing patterns, particularly during sleep (Closs, 1994; De Conno & Foley, 1995). However, it is not necessary to withold opioids automatically if such patterns are identified.

Healthcare professionals are often worried that respiratory depression may kill a patient, particularly when the dose of opioid is increased rapidly or when patients are in the terminal phase of their illness (De Conno & Foley, 1995). Some professionals are unaccustomed to the very large doses of opioids which are employed to relieve pain in patients with cancer and may be very uncomfortable with giving an equivalent dose of parenteral analgesic to a patient who is no longer able to take oral medication. This may be because they are concerned that the administration of parenteral opioids to a dying patient may create some ambiguity about the cause of death. This was certainly the situation in the case reported by Peate (1996). Some sound advice has been offered by Henkelman (1994) who recommends that given our knowledge of respiratory depression associated with opioid administration, the nurse must balance the known and predictable beneficial effects against the unlikely and reversible harmful effects.

Misconceptions about the placebo response

Improvements in a patient's pain can be brought about for three different reasons. First, the self-limiting nature of some pains and fluctuating nature of others means that many pains will improve with time. Secondly, therapeutic interventions may ameliorate pain; and finally, non-specific effects of treatment may lead some patients to report improvements in their pain (Turner *et al.*, 1994). Non-specific effects of treatment are often seen following the administration of a placebo.

A placebo is an intervention designed to simulate medical therapy or nursing care, but not believed by healthcare professionals to be therapeutic for a particular condition (Turner *et al.*, 1994). Placebo also refers to inactive substances packaged to appear to be active medication. Placebo drugs are usually encountered in clinical trials where their use allows active drugs to be compared to 'nothing' in an unbiased way – everybody is receiving a tablet of the same appearance.

Placebo effects can be extremely powerful and often will act in a synergistic way with specific treatment effects to bring about an improvement in a patient's condition. Unfortunately these impressive effects are often misinterpreted by healthcare professionals as an indication that the patient is lying about their pain or that the pain is 'all in the head'. Such interpretations demonstrate a lack of insight into the factors which influence the placebo response (Table 5.4) and can result in unethical behaviours. For example, some healthcare professionals who think that a patient's expressions of pain is excessive or unnecessary will withhold analgesics or administer a placebo medication (Bond, 1980). Others would reduce the analgesic or give a placebo when their patients complain that their last dose of analgesic did not completely relieve their pain and that they continue to experience severe pain (Cohen, 1980). Some readers may feel that the above mentioned studies are quite old and that the prevalence of placebo pill or injection use is uncommon in clinical practice today. However, the US Oncology Nursing Society (ONS) was so concerned about the widespread use of placebos that it recently published a position paper recommending that nurses should not use placebos in the assessment and management of cancer pain even if there is a medical order to do so (McCaffrey *et al.*, 1996).

Table 5.4 Factors influencing the placebo response.

- Patient and healthcare professional's expectation of treatment effect.
- Enthusiastic administration of a drug.
- Patient's perception of the level of expertise of healthcare professional.
- Reputation, expense and impressiveness of treatment.
- Healthcare professional showing a warm, sympathetic, interested attitude towards patient.
- Level of patient anxiety.

It is a serious violation of a nurse's code of ethics to administer a placebo in order to legitimise a belief that a patient is a malingerer or that the pain is not real. If discovered, such deception will invariably result in a loss of trust and will damage the relationship between the patient and the healthcare team. In this era of accountability for practice and as a result of the upsurge in medical litigation, it is unlikely that such practices will survive in the future. Nevertheless, it is important to challenge the misconceptions people hold about placebo responses in order to ensure that the inappropriate use of placebos becomes extinct sooner rather than later.

Ageism

The incidence of acute and chronic pain is highest in elderly people. It is ironic that an elderly person's pain is more likely to be undertreated than that of a younger counterpart (Closs, 1994). Ageism, which can be defined as stereotyping and prejudice against old age (Butler, 1975), is thought to be one of the reasons why elderly patients' pain is so poorly managed

(Harkins *et al.*, 1990; Jacox *et al.*, 1994). A number of misconceptions exist about pain in the elderly including beliefs that elderly people have decreased pain sensitivity and increased pain tolerance. Moreover, opioids are often not prescribed for, or administered to, elderly patients because of exaggerated fears of side effects such as respiratory depression, or because staff are less likely to believe an elderly patient's report of pain (Closs, 1996). Finally, many people assume that pain is part of the normal ageing process, which may result in the pain being ignored or inadequate assessment and treatment.

It is interesting to note that, in the context of pain, elderly people are not the only group confronted by ageist attitudes. For years it was thought that young children, especially neonates, could not experience pain the way adults do (Friedrichs *et al.*, 1995) and that they were more easily addicted to opioids (Liebeskind & Melzack, 1987). As a result children are often given less analgesics than adults, and invasive procedures are often carried out on them without adequate analgesia (Schechter *et al.*, 1986; Southall *et al.*, 1993). Until recently, it was standard practice to carry out surgical procedures on neonates using paralytic agents alone, without anaesthesia (Friedrichs *et al.*, 1995). This was based on the belief that an infant could not feel pain because of an immature nervous system. The current thinking is that neonates and infants do feel pain, that pain may actually be harmful to a developing nervous system and that younger children may be more sensitive to pain than older children (Shandor Miles & Neelon, 1989; Bozzette, 1993; McCaffrey & Beebe, 1994).

As Liebeskind and Melzack (1987) have stated, it is appalling '...that pain is most poorly managed in those most defenceless against it – the young and the elderly.' Clearly more work is required to banish ageist attitudes from modern healthcare. An important step towards achieving this goal would be the eradication of the many myths surrounding the management of pain in elderly and young patients.

5.2 Factors related to patients and their families

Reluctance to report pain

Patients and their carers also contribute to the problem of poor pain management. A major barrier to the effective management of pain is patients' reluctance to report pain (Ward & Gatwood, 1994). There may be many reasons for this. Fears of addiction and the side effects of pain medication may cause some people to be hesitant in reporting pain (Francke & Theeuwen, 1994). Patients may believe that their pain is inevitable and may be fatalistic about the benefits of analgesics, so they end up saying 'why bother reporting my pain, nothing is going to work anyway' (Yates *et al.*, 1995). Some patients may suffer in silence because they believe that 'good' patients do not complain of pain and should not bother their caregivers (Francke & Theeuwen, 1994; Yates *et al.*, 1995), whereas others believe that complaining about their pain may distract their doctor from the more important task of treating their disease. In contrast, some patients do not like to talk about their pain with people whom they consider to be total strangers, and others stop complaining of pain because they are faced with a situation over which they believe they have little control (Meinhart & McCaffrey, 1983).

Ward and Gatwood (1994), who also found that people shared similar concerns and misconceptions about pain and its management, recommend that educational programmes should be run for the general public with the purpose of dispelling myths about the use of opioid analgesics. Moreover, they recommend that during a patient's first encounter with a healthcare professional, efforts are made to reinforce the message that pain can be relieved.

In some cultures, a stoic reaction to pain is strongly valued and public expressions of pain are generally frowned upon (Garro, 1990). There would be a social stigma associated with reporting pain which may cause people from such cultures to refrain from complaining of pain and 'put on a brave face'. A British study found that this behaviour was so admired by nursing staff that it was rewarded by the administration of pain-relieving medication (Bond, 1980). Culture is not the only determinant of stoical reactions to pain. Men are often socialised to believe that pain is a test of manhood and therefore they should remain stoical in the face of pain (Wall & Jones, 1991).

To some people pain has a high moral value which means that they are often willing to endure great pain (see Chapter 4). For example, according to Catholic doctrine purgatory is a place of spiritual purging and temporary suffering before accession into heaven, where one feels no pain or suffering. Spiritual purging is necessary to cleanse the soul of sins committed in the past. One of the authors (KR) comes from a culture where the Catholic church is the predominant religion and some of her patients have said that they viewed their pain as their 'purgatory on earth' and the endurance of that pain would benefit them in their life after death. Many people do not subscribe to such doctrine, but for those that do, it may mean that they choose to hold on to their pain and do not report it.

Non-compliance with treatment

Non-compliance with pain medication can be a significant problem (Austin *et al.*, 1986; Snelling, 1994; Ward & Gatwood, 1994). This may be because patients do not understand the instructions about how to take their analgesics (Niven, 1989), which is often a reflection of poor information giving on the part of healthcare professionals (see discussion in Chaper 4). A patient may be also non-compliant with their medication because of misconceptions and fears about their treatment. Austin *et al.* (1986) found that 50% of terminally ill cancer patients with severe pain had not followed all aspects of their prescribed analgesic regimen. This occurred despite the provision of regular support and education from hospice homecare staff. Patients indicated that there were two main reasons for their non-compliance – first, fear of addiction and secondly a desire to maintain personal control over their present situation. Some patients said that they wanted to 'feel the pain' so that they would know that they were still alive. The authors suggest that, at a time of such huge loss, the act of determining their own pain medication regimen may give patients a feeling of control. Patients may also have chosen not to comply with their analgesic regimen because they fear that tolerance will develop and that there will be no 'pain killer' available when the pain gets really bad.

A family caregiver is often the person in charge of the administration of pain medication in a homecare setting. Some caregivers may try to limit the amount of analgesics used because of their own or the patients' fear of addiction, tolerance, or respiratory depression (Ferrell *et al.*, 1991). This problem is further compounded by the fact that family caregivers rarely receive instruction in the use of both pharmacological and non-pharmacological pain relief methods. The use of denial as a coping mechanism can further complicate the situation, resulting in a scenario where both the patient and family ignore the patient's pain, because to acknowledge the pain would mean having to acknowledge that the disease might be progressing. A pain education programme may help improve family caregivers' knowledge and attitudes regarding pain management (Ferrell *et al.*, 1995).

Patients may not disclose to health professionals the exact amount of analgesics they are taking. Snelling (1994) provides some excellent examples of situations where patients take more than the prescribed amount of medication and then collude with their partners to keep this information from the healthcare professionals involved in their care. Clearly such a scenario could result in doctors making inaccurate decisions about what analgesics to prescribe and, as a result, patients may experience greater side effects from their medications.

5.3 Factors within the healthcare system

Barriers to opioid availability

A very important barrier to achieving effective pain control is that some analgesics are not available in many countries (Report of a Subcommittee on Palliative Care, 1993). Moreover, in some countries there is widespread reluctance to use strong opioids. In nearly half the countries of the world there is little or no use of morphine (Joranson, 1993). Statistics issued by the International Narcotics Control Board (1991) have revealed that 87% of the morphine available for medicinal use worldwide is used by only 20 developed countries. The top 10 consumers of morphine worldwide used 57% of the world supply (see Table 5.5). A number of barriers to the use of morphine have been identified and include:

- constraints on availability of drugs as a result of government efforts to combat the illicit use of drugs;
- restrictive laws and regulations which interfere with the opioid production and distribution;
- archaic prescribing regulations;
- poor medical, nursing and pharmacy practices (United Nations, 1989).

Table 5.5 Countries with the highest consumption of morphine (in alphabetical order). Statistics issued by the International Narcotics Control Board (1991).

- Australia
- Canada
- Denmark
- Iceland
- Ireland
- New Zealand
- Norway
- Sweden
- United Kingdom
- United States

In many countries of the European Union the use of opioids is obstructed by restrictive prescribing laws (Zenz & Willweber-Strumpf, 1993). With some notable exceptions, special prescription forms or books are required, which increases the bureaucracy associated with prescribing opioids. The short validity of prescriptions in some countries has the potential to interfere with the patient's quality of life. For example, many patients would not be able to go away on holidays for longer than a few days. According to Zenz & Willweber-Strumpf (1993) many of these prescribing regulations date from World War II when the authorities were very concerned about preventing the illicit trafficking of drugs. At this time there was little or no understanding of the benefits of opioids in the management of pain. These laws have not changed in the face of more enlightened thinking about the use of opioids, and clearly they have huge potential to obstruct the effective management of chronic pain, particularly cancer pain. There seems to be a fear that the liberalisation of prescribing regulations will result in an increase in illicit drug use or drug trafficking.

This situation may actually be made worse if a EU directive requiring doctors to use special prescriptions for drugs covered under the UN Single Convention on Narcotic Drugs (1961, amended 1972) is enforced (Commission of the European Communities, 1990). Unfortunately, the use of multiple-copy prescription programmes may mean that healthcare professionals '. . . may be reluctant to prescribe, stock or dispense opioids as they feel that there is a possibility of their professional licences being suspended or revoked by the governing authority in cases where large quantities of opioids are provided to an individual, even though the medical need for such drugs can be proved' (World Health Organisation, 1990).

Patients living in the community may experience some difficulty in getting their prescriptions filled. Pharmacies in urban areas, particularly inner city areas, may be reluctant to stock large amounts of opioids because of the risk of theft. On the other hand, pharmacies in rural areas may not stock opioids because there is little demand for them. The overall result is that patients may be faced with a significant delay in getting their pain medication. In hospitals gaining easy access to sufficient stocks of opioids is rarely problematic; however, considerable delays in administration can occur because of the policy that opioids should be checked by two nurses before they are administered (White, 1985). Nurses may make a deliberate attempt to delay this process further if they misinterpret a patient's request for opioids as a sign that the patient is addicted (Alleyne & Thomas, 1994).

Joranson (1993) argues that healthcare professionals need to understand the drug regulatory system in their own country so that they will be better prepared to take action to address barriers to opioid availability. Otherwise we may find that in our own country, 'overly restrictive approaches may, in the end, merely result in depriving a majority of the population access to opiate medications' (United Nations, 1989). An increase in the medicinal use of opioids does not automatically mean that the illicit use of opioids will increase. This message needs to be conveyed to both the people who legislate for opioid use and the general public alike.

Breakdown in continuity of care

The system of organising nursing work may pose some problems in terms of achieving optimal pain control. Many hospital units use some form of patient allocation as a means of organising nursing work. Others have adopted a system of Primary Nursing. These systems mean that a smaller number of nurses are involved in the care of a smaller number of patients. Nurses have greater opportunity to get to know their patients and to carry out more in-depth assessments. Patients themselves recommend such systems as a means of improving the management of pain (Copp, 1990). As one patient in Copp's (1990) study explained, 'I'd like one doctor and nurse each shift. There isn't enough energy to describe the pain over and over again.'

This situation is the ideal, but the reality is that, for economic reasons, the emphasis is on discharging patients into the community as soon as possible (White, 1985). The turnover of patients is very high and nurses have little opportunity to build up any sort of relationship with their patients. In addition, shorter working weeks, an increase in the use of part-time staff and holidays mean that there is an increased flow of nurses through the wards. Thus, even with Primary Nursing or some form of patient allocation, there is no guarantee that patients will have a small group of nurses involved in their care for the duration of their stay.

In the community it is much easier to achieve some degree of continuity of care. However, fragmentation of care can occur due to a lack of communication between the hospital and those caring for patients in the community. This problem can be exacerbated when a patient is being seen by a number of different doctors and moving between a number of different healthcare settings, and no one person is willing to take responsibility for the overall management of the patient's pain. Some would suggest that this situation occurs because such a low priority is given to the management of pain (Fagerhaugh & Strauss, 1977; Sofaer, 1992; Jacox *et al.*, 1994). The Report of the Royal Colleges of Surgeons and Anaesthetists (1990) recommends that a named member of staff should be responsible for a hospital policy on pain management. This may help overcome the problem of lack of accountability.

Another impediment to the effective management of pain is the lack of specialised pain management services which could provide advice for those dealing with complex pain problems. This problem has been addressed by bodies such as the Royal Colleges of Surgeons and Anaesthetists (1990) who recommended that acute pain services be established as a matter of urgency. A number of hospitals have responded to this recommendation by establishing such a service; however, this is not widespread and much more effort is required to rectify this situation. The establishment of both hospital and community based palliative care teams has contributed greatly to the improved management of pain in patients with advanced cancer; however, as with acute pain, more services are required. In order to improve this situation further the World Health Organisation (1996) has recommended that more resources be allocated to cancer pain relief and palliative care. It could be argued that patients with chronic non-malignant pain are least served by the present services, and special efforts are required in order to meet the diverse and complex needs of this patient population.

5.4 Concluding remarks

The evidence is clear – a considerable number of patients continue to experience unnecessary pain. A multitude of factors maintain this situation which means that it will be extremely difficult to bring about any meaningful change. Nevertheless, we should not be deterred from this onerous task. An important first step is an attempt to improve the knowledge of both healthcare professionals and the general public about the nature of pain and its treatments. This may go some way towards eradicating the many prevailing myths and misconceptions about pain and opioids in society today. It is also important to think of pain and its treatments in more global terms – the healthcare system and bureaucratic laws are significant barriers to the effective management of pain. There is no good reason for depriving those who need opioid analgesics of these agents. Policies and legislation should be scrutinised carefully to ensure that they are not creating such a situation. As the control of distressing symptoms falls more into the domain of nursing practice, it is nurses who should address many of the problems raised in this chapter.

Summary of Chapter 5

- Despite the fact that we have both the means and the knowledge to ameliorate pain effectively, a significant number of patients still experience unacceptable levels of pain.
- Both nurses and doctors possess poor levels of knowledge about pain and its management, and many health professionals indicate that they feel ill prepared to care for patients in pain.
- Nurses' perceptions of patient pain is often quite different from those of their patient.
- Pain assessment is often compromised by inadequate and inaccurate data collection and interpretion and pain assessment tools are rarely used by nurses in their everyday clinical practice.
- Information about the patient's pain is often recorded incompletely and inconsistently.
- Fear of addiction on the part of health professionals is arguably the most important reason why pain is so poorly managed. This situation is made worse by the fact that patients and their families share similar fears about addiction.
- Confusion exists about the definition of addiction, tolerance and physical dependence.
- A fear of respiratory depression is prevalent amongst healthcare professionals, particularly in relation to terminally-ill and elderly patients.
- Healthcare professionals often misinterpret a placebo response as meaning that the patient is lying about his or her pain or that the pain is psychogenic in origin; placebos should never be used to legitimise a belief that the patient is a malingerer or that the pain is not real.
- Pain is often poorly managed in elderly patients and young children.
- A major barrier to the effective management of pain is patients' reluctance to report pain because of beliefs that the pain is inevitable or the wish to be a 'good' patient; some people are willing to endure pain because they see it as having a high moral value.
- Non-compliance with treatment can contribute to poor pain control.
- Restrictive prescribing laws and bureaucracy surrounding the storage and administration of opioids can deprive patients of easy access to opioids at a time when they most need them.
- An increase in the medicinal use of opioids does not automatically mean that the illicit use of opioids will increase.
- Any factor which interferes with nurses' ability to build up relationships with their patients may pose problems in terms of achieving optimal pain control.
- Breakdowns in continuity of care can occur when a patient is being seen by a number of different doctors across a number of healthcare settings.

Chapter 6

The Nursing Management of Patients with Pain

Most nurses will be called upon regularly to make clinical decisions about pain. Some of these decisions will be relatively clear-cut, but others will be highly complex. We have already identified the fact that nurses often make poor clinical decisions when caring for people experiencing pain (see Chapter 5). Clearly there are a number of reasons why this occurs. An important, and often overlooked, reason is the uncertain nature of the clinical decision making process (Pellegrino, 1979). Nurses use a number of different decision making strategies to overcome this uncertainty (Baumann & Deber, 1989). Unfortunately these strategies are not foolproof and do not protect nurses from making poor decisions for which, ultimately, they are accountable (UKCC, 1992; Watson, 1995). This chapter identifies ways in which nurses can make better clinical decisions when caring for patients in pain.

6.1 Pain assessment

A good assessment is pivotal to the successful management of any distressing symptom. If the causes of a patient's symptom are not clearly identified, it will be impossible to make decisions about which interventions are most appropriate for that particular patient. Patients can experience many different types of pain (see Chapter 3) and each of these pains warrant slightly different approaches to assessment and management. In addition, assessment has an important role in identifying the patient at risk of developing pain. Patients who fall into this category include those about to undergo some type of invasive procedure, those who have received some treatment which causes painful side effects and those who have a chronic, progressive disease such as cancer or arthritis.

For many years it has been acknowledged that the patient's own expression of symptom intensity is the 'gold standard' in assessment (McCaffrey, 1980). However, such unidimensional assessment can result in misuse of pharmacological and non-pharmacological interventions (Bruera & Watanabe, 1994). Recently, it has become evident that a multi-dimensional approach to assessment is required. This allows for the identification of the various factors which might be influencing the patient's perception and expression of pain. If these factors are identified, the nurse will be in a better position to determine realistic goals and decide on the various measures necessary to achieve optimal control of pain.

Assessment strategies

A number of different strategies are used to assess the person in pain. The most important of these strategies is effective communication. This is particularly important for patients with chronic pain who may have been living with that pain for many years. They are experts on their own pain and therefore should be given the opportunity to indicate, not only how intense their pain is but also what it means to them, the extent to which it is impacting on their lives and the strategies they have employed to cope with the situation (Arathuzik, 1991). Many authors have pointed out how important it is to listen to the patient (Saunders, 1988; Copp, 1974), to ask clear, unambiguous questions of the patient (Carr, 1990) and to believe what the patient says (McCaffrey, 1980). Communication can be fraught with difficulty, not least because a pain experience can 'actively destroy' language making it impossible for patients to convey the reality of that experience (Scarry, 1985). A number of other factors interfere with communication including:

- patients' reluctance to discuss their pain;
- lack of continuity in nurse-patient relationships;
- healthcare professionals' use of blocking verbal behaviours;
- patients' inability to express themselves due to cognitive impairment, lack of vocabulary, excessive body weakness or a speaking impediment;
- patients' inability to speak the language spoken by their carers;
- hearing impediments.

As a consequence, information on the patient's pain, on which nurses base their clinical decisions, is often incomplete and therefore, easily misinterpreted (see Chapter 5 for a more complete discussion on this issue).

Observation and measurement are also important assessment strategies. As previously mentioned, patients in pain may manifest a number of different behaviours which provide important clues about a person's pain (Wilkie *et al.*, 1989). Observing pain behaviours is particularly important when assessing pain in people who are cognitively impaired or in those who either lack, or have limited, ability to communicate verbally. It should be remembered, however, that overt behaviours do not always constitute direct expressions of intensity or quality of the pain experience (Sutters & Miaskowski, 1992). There is a difference between pain expression behaviours and pain control behaviours, and it is important to clarify with patients the reason why they are manifesting a particular behaviour – otherwise behaviours may be misinterpreted (Wilkie *et al.*,1989). A discussion on the measurement of pain will follow later on in this chapter.

When a patient presents with pain, a number of facts should be established as soon as possible (Table 6.1). In addition, patients should be asked what they think is causing their pain. It is important at this stage to note what words patients use to describe their pain. Some patients will not use the word 'pain', but use words such as 'heaviness', 'discomfort', 'unpleasant feeling' instead. Whatever word the patient uses should be employed in subsequent assessments. A physical examination should be carried out to determine whether there are any local signs of inflammation or abnormality (e.g. tenderness, guarding, swelling) which would give an indication of the cause of the pain. The patient may be experiencing a number of different types of pain and the above mentioned facts need to be established for each pain.

Table 6.1 Factors to be established when the patient first presents with pain.

- Intensity
- Location
- Onset
- Duration
- Quality (e.g. burning, aching, stabbing, etc.)
- Prodromal symptoms (e.g. restlessness, uneasiness, etc.)
- Aggravating factors
- Alleviating factors
- Variations in pain over time
- Associated symptoms (e.g. nausea)

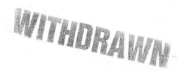

Patients' perceptions of pain severity are often associated with their perception of the impact that pain has on their daily life (Arathuzik, 1991), and therefore information about this important aspect needs to be collected. Pain can cause difficulties with sleep, nutrition, concentration, mobility, and activity. Restrictions in activity for even a short period of time can result in the patient experiencing fatigue (Winningham *et al.*, 1994). As a result patients may find themselves in a vicious cycle of having to decrease their activity because of their pain and then becoming easily exhausted when they attempt even moderate activity. This may mean that the patient is unable to continue to work, which in turn may lead to financial insecurity. In addition, patients may be less likely to make the effort to socialise which may cause them to experience loneliness.

The degree to which pain has impacted on the family should be assessed. It is important to identify whether the pain condition has caused any strain in family relationships and how supportive the family are of the patient. Dysfunctional family relationships can facilitate the patient to develop maladaptive pain behaviours (Snelling, 1994), and the degree to which this is occurring should be evaluated.

The names of all the prescription and over-the-counter analgesics the patient is currently taking should be noted, as should the level of pain relief associated with each agent. It is also important to check whether the patient has been compliant with the analgesic regimen and if the patient has experienced any side effects from the medications. The patient may hold negative attitudes towards opioid analgesics, a particular route of delivery of analgesic agents (e.g. rectal or parenteral) or towards the use of supportive techniques, such as massage; and it is useful to establish the patient's attitude at an early stage. There are contraindications associated with the use of some analgesic agents. For example, aspirin should not be given to thrombocytopenic patients because it can increase the risk of bleeding, nor to children under 12 years of age (Wilkes *et al.*, 1994). The presence of any condition which would prevent the use of certain analgesic agents should be noted.

A number of different factors influence a person's perception and expression of pain (see Chapter 4). In making assessments, it is important to be aware of these factors and to establish the degree to which they are influencing the patient's perception and expression of pain at this time. For example, if patients lack confidence about the ability of the healthcare team to control pain they may be reluctant to report their pain (Francke & Theeuwen, 1994; Ward & Gatwood, 1994). These factors should also be assessed in the person at risk of developing pain. Patients may be frightened or apprehensive about undergoing an invasive procedure if they have had a negative experience previously with that particular procedure (Scott, 1994). Having an expectation of a negative pain experience may cause a person to experience more pain (Garro, 1990). Many of the factors which contribute to the person's pain experience will only become apparent as the nurse builds up a trusting relationship with the patient, which may take a considerable amount of time. This highlights the fact that assessment is not a once-off event – new information is continuously becoming available and decisions often need to be changed in the light of new information.

Patients in chronic pain often use numerous different coping strategies to deal with their pain, including:

- taking medication;
- positioning themselves in a certain way;
- distraction;
- pressure manipulation;
- heat and cold (Wilkie *et al.*, 1989);
- cognitive reinterpretation;
- relaxation and visualisation (Arathuzik, 1991).

Information should be collected about which strategies the patient has been using and how effective the strategies have been. Some strategies, such as restrictive positioning, may actually cause the patient more problems in the long term, whereas other strategies can be very beneficial in dealing with the pain. When a beneficial strategy is identified, it should be documented and incorporated into the patient's plan of care.

6.2 Pain measurement

Pain is a subjective experience and as such can only be quantified indirectly. Many attempts have been made to develop measurement tools which would provide objective data about different dimensions of the pain experience. This has occurred for a number of different reasons. Healthcare professionals often have difficulty in accepting the statement that 'pain is whatever the experiencing person says it is' (McCaffrey 1980). Measurement tools provide a valuable means of overcoming this problem since they provide objective data, which is then documented, making it very difficult for healthcare professionals to ignore. For the same reason measurement tools provide an important means of maintaining continuity of care. This is particularly important in the care of patients with chronic pain where it is common to have involvement from a large number of health professionals, often in different care settings. This situation can lead to breakdowns in communication and discrepancies in opinion about the patient's pain. The objective information provided by measurement tools helps to determine the effectiveness of various interventions. Finally, measurement tools provide important data to substantiate or refute the effectiveness of analgesic agents which are being tested in clinical trials.

A number of valid and reliable tools are available to measure pain, as set out in the following section. Each of these tools has advantages and disadvantages, and any data collected should be interpreted in the light of a particular tool's limitations.

Pain rating scales

Pain intensity can be measured using a number of different types of rating scales (Figure 6.1). Verbal rating scales (VRSs) are category scales consisting of various words, such as mild or severe, which are thought to indicate the intensity of pain. The words are placed in rank order at equal intervals along a line. Some authors have questioned whether there is equal spacing between the various categories (Sriwatanakul *et al.*, 1983). An additional problem is that patients have to put their pain experiences into words which might not necessarily describe those experiences. The advantage of VRSs lies in their ease of administration and scoring.

A Visual Analogue Scale (VAS) consists of a 10 cm line anchored at each end with words such as 'no pain' and 'the worst pain possible'. The line may be either vertical or horizontal. Patients are asked to place a mark at the

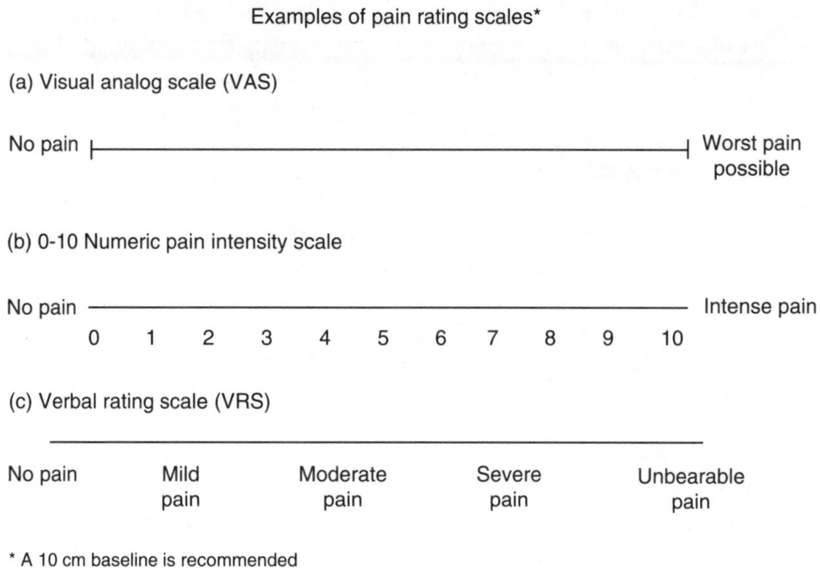

Examples of pain rating scales*

(a) Visual analog scale (VAS)

No pain |———————————————————————————————————| Worst pain
possible

(b) 0-10 Numeric pain intensity scale

No pain ——————————————————————————————————— Intense pain

   0   1   2   3   4   5   6   7   8   9   10

(c) Verbal rating scale (VRS)

No pain	Mild pain	Moderate pain	Severe pain	Unbearable pain

* A 10 cm baseline is recommended

Figure 6.1 Verbal rating scales (VRSs) and visual analogue scales (VASs) used to measure pain.

point on the line which best represents their experience of pain. A VAS with numbers placed along the line is referred to as Numeric Pain Intensity Scale. A VAS places few demands on sick patients and is sensitive to changes in pain intensity (Choiniere *et al.*, 1990; Melzack & Katz, 1994). While most people have little difficulty understanding how to use VAS (Chapman *et al.*, 1985), some authors have argued that people may find the concept hard to understand (Huskisson, 1983). This highlights the importance of providing a clear explanation to the patient. Unfortunately, this can add greatly to the time taken to administer a VAS which diminishes one of its most important strengths (Schofield, 1995). The disadvantage of these rating scales is that they only measure one dimension of pain. Great care needs to be taken when comparing studies which have employed either a VRS or a VAS for data collection, as there is little consistency in the words used or in the way the line is drawn (Deschamps *et al.*, 1988). A VRS has been shown to be less sensitive than a VAS, especially to changes in mild pain (Deschamps *et al.*, 1988). Moreover, a VAS is thought to reflect more precisely changes in the intensity of the pain experiences (Ohnhaus & Adler, 1975).

Body diagrams

Body diagrams facilitate the documentation of the location and distribution of a patient's pain. This is particularly important with cancer pain, as the patient may be experiencing pain at a number of different sites. Body diagrams can either by filled in by the clinician or the patient. Additional information about the pain, such as an indication of the area which hurts the most, can be included on the diagram. In children this can be achieved by getting them to colour the body diagram with a colour which represents for them different levels of pain. This can also provide useful information about changes in pain intensity over time (Eland, 1985).

The advantage of body diagrams is that they are easy to use and provide clear evidence of the extent and sites of pain. Their disadvantage lies in the fact that they measure a very limited part of the pain experience. For this reason body diagrams are often incorporated into pain questionnaires such as the McGill Pain Questionnaire and the London Hospital Pain Observation Chart (Raiman, 1986).

Pain questionnaires

Pain questionnaires employ a combination of different approaches, such as open and closed questions, rating scales and body diagrams to measure different dimensions of the pain experience. A number of these questionnaires are available including:

- McGill Pain Questionnaire (Melzack, 1975);
- Wisconsin Brief Pain Questionnaire (Daut *et al.*, 1983);
- The London Hospital Pain Observation Chart (Raiman, 1986);
- Edmonton Symptom Assessment System (Bruera *et al.*, 1991);
- Initial Pain-Assessment Tool (McCaffrey & Beebe, 1994).

The McGill Pain Questionnaire (MPQ), probably the most well known of the above questionnaires, measures the sensory, affective and evaluative dimensions of the pain experience (Melzack & Katz, 1994). In addition, the MPQ measures present pain intensity, assesses the pattern of the pain and contains a line drawing of the body to show the location of the pain(s). A short-form MPQ (SF-MPQ) has been developed for use in situations where time to collect information is limited (Melzack, 1987). The MPQ takes between 2 and 10 minutes to administer depending on which form is being used. It is thought to be one of the most adequate and useful instruments available for measuring pain (McGuire, 1992). A major advantage of the MPQ is that it is a reliable and valid measure of multiple dimensions of pain. Both forms of the instrument can discriminate between different types of pain and can demonstrate the effect of treatment on pain. Another possible advantage of the MPQ is that it incorporates an extensive list of words which people use to describe different aspects of their pain experience. The provision of such an extensive vocabulary of pain can be helpful for patients because it facilitates them to describe their pain when they themselves cannot find the appropriate words.

The MPQ also has a number of disadvantages. In comparison to a VAS or a VRS, the MPQ is time consuming to complete and requires more concentration, which may make it unsuitable to use with very sick people. The SF-MPQ offers a potential means of overcoming this problem, although its usefulness with very sick patients in a variety of clinical settings has yet to be demonstrated. Another problem associated with the MPQ is that some of the words used may not be understood by all patients (Chapman *et al.*, 1985; Deschamps *et al.*, 1988).

Observational charts

It is possible to measure pain objectively by observing and quantifying behaviours which accompany pain such as use of medication, level of functioning and non-verbal pain expression (Bonnel & Boureau, 1985; Chapman *et al.*, 1985). This approach is especially useful for providing an objective measure of pain in children or adults who have a poor command of the language, or in confused patients (Melzack & Katz, 1994). One such scale that has been developed is the discomfort scale for patients with dementia of the Alzheimer type (DS-DAT) (Wells, 1990; Hurley, 1992). This scale measures a number of behaviours such as breathing, vocalisation, facial expression, type of body language and amount of fidgeting. It is not thought to measure pain accurately, although it does provide an accurate measure of discomfort (Closs, 1995).

The major disadvantage of observing patients' behaviours is that their opinion about their pain is not sought directly. Furthermore, as has been discussed in Chapter 4, many factors affect a person's expression of pain. As Le Resche and Dworkin (1984) point out, it is a mistake to assume that pain is always 'written all over the face'. It should be remembered that much of the behaviour being measured may not be an accurate indicator of pain in all people.

Pain diaries

Another way of recording pain behaviours is to ask patients to keep a pain diary. These diaries, which come in either paper or electronic form, usually collect information about the severity of the patient's pain and mood, plus details of any medication taken and activities undertaken. The advantages of patients using pain diaries are that they enable patients to be more active participants in their own care, they can provide useful information about the impact of pain on a person's life over a period of time without fear of recall bias and, finally, diaries provide information on the effectiveness of pain medication. Nevertheless, there are some drawbacks associated with the use of pain diaries. The mere fact of having to record pain frequently in a diary may focus patients' attention unnecessarily on to their pain. However, there is some new evidence available to demonstrate that this is not necessarily the case (Cruise *et al.*, 1996). Another problem with pain diaries is that patients sometimes provide inaccurate information when reporting activities which needs to be kept in mind when interpreting the information recorded (Chapman *et al.*, 1985).

Practical aspects of pain measurement

Unfortunately measurement tools are still not an accepted part of nursing practice, possibly because they are not routinely included in the standard nursing observation chart (Scott, 1994). More and more healthcare professionals are becoming aware of the advantages of using measurement tools and are starting to use these tools in their everyday clinical practice. The decision about which instrument to use in a particular clinical setting is based on a number of different considerations. To be useful an instrument should be: multidimensional; valid; reliable; sensitive; easy to administer; and not place undue demands on the nurse or patient (Schofield, 1995).

If these conditions are met, it is more likely that the instrument chosen will be used. It is probably a good idea to have a small number of different measurement tools available for use in particular situations. In this instance, staff need to be careful to use the same measurement tool with a particular patient, otherwise inconsistent information may be collected. It is also important to remember that pain in different sites should be assessed independently since there could be different causes for each pain. Selection of a measurement tool for an individual patient will depend on a number of factors including:

- level of pain during assessment;
- the complexity of the pain;
- patient's general condition;
- patient's level of concentration;
- patient's cognitive ability;
- patient's command of the language.

In some instances, such as when the patient is in extreme pain, it is clearly inappropriate to use a measurement tool, in others a short assessment tool will provide the information required. For patients with chronic pain it is invariably appropriate to use a more comprehensive measurement tool which will help to provide a more complete picture of the total pain experience. It is sometimes useful to obtain multiple measures of pain using a number of different tools. Regardless of which measurement tools are in use, it is important to remember that since pain is a subjective experience, the patient's own report of pain remains a very important measure of that experience. This report should be regarded as valid as indirect measures of pain. However, it is important to acknowledge that in some rare instances, such as when patients have secondary gains from their pain, some caution should be exercised when interpreting patients' self-reports of pain.

6.3 Preventing errors during assessment

It has been emphasised already in this chapter that a good assessment is the cornerstone in the management of any distressing symptom. Unfortunately, it is often quite difficult to make a good assessment, which means that it is not uncommon for poor or incorrect diagnostic decisions to be made. The inevitable result of this is that poor decisions are made about which interventions are required. There are a number of sources of error in the diagnostic process including:

- failing to collect critical information (e.g. patient's viewpoint);
- collecting inaccurate information;
- making assumptions without clarifying their validity;
- stereotyping and making generalisations about patients on the basis of their culture, race, sex, age, non-conformist behaviour, etc.;
- making decisions too quickly;
- overestimating the probability of a rare or impressive event;
- lacking clinical knowledge or experience (Gordon 1987; Iyer *et al.*, 1995).

Moreover, human beings are often loathe to change decisions once they have been made, despite the fact that there may be evidence available which indicates that their decisions might be incorrect (Gordon, 1987). It is important that nurses become aware of their own particular biases in decision making and seek ways of avoiding these biases in practice.

A number of factors may facilitate nurses to make better assessments. Clinical algorithms such as those developed by Walker *et al.* (1990) (see Figure 6.2) and Gould *et al.* (1992) provide guidelines on the type of information which should be collected when assessing pain. Such algorithms are particularly useful as guides for less-experienced and knowledgeable staff.

The system of organising nursing work can either inhibit or facilitate the assessment process. Continuity in the nurse-patient relationship is greatly facilitated by the system known as Primary Nursing (Manthey, 1992). In this system the nurse is given total responsibility for the care of a particular patient for the duration of that patient's hospital stay. This means that nurses are given the opportunity of building up more in-depth relationships with their patients, and therefore it is more likely that patients will provide their nurses with pertinent information about their pain. The nurse is also in a better position to monitor changes in the patient's pain experience. It seems clear, however, that regardless of which system of organising nursing work is in use, the nurse's ability to communicate effectively will have an enormous influence on the quality of information which is collected during assessment.

HOW IS THE PATIENT COPING?

WELL	WITH DIFFICULTY, OR POORLY
Patient feels calm, contented, confident, in control	Patient feels: ANXIOUS: worried, frightened, unsure, tense DEPRESSED: low self esteem, helpless, hopeless, guilty or suicidal RESENTFUL: bitter, angry, irritable LONELY COMPLAINS A LOT

Provide supportive visits to give encouragement and maintain confidence

DOES THE PATIENT THINK THAT THE PAIN IS UNDER CONTROL?

YES	NO
Annoying or troublesome, but mostly under control	Pain is miserable, intense, unbearable, frightening, punishing, cruel, vicious

Assess levels of least and worst pain. Encourage judicious use of analgesics when necessary.
Identify and encourage avoidance of trigger factors.
Encourage, provide, teach, alternative active pain-controlling strategies for patient's own use.
Monitor pain-relieving, and iatrogenic effects of all drugs.

DOES THE PATIENT FEEL WELL-INFORMED ABOUT THE ILLNESS OR PAINFUL CONDITION?

YES	NO
Fully informed or unconcerned	Wishes to know results of tests, cause or potential outcome of present condition

Provide information and feedback.
Involve patient in assessing and monitoring progress.
Refer to GP for information where necessary.
Put in touch with self-help groups.

DOES THE PATIENT FEEL OCCUPIED?

YES	NO
Involved in self-care, social or recreational activities	Feels useless, little or nothing to do

Encourage carers to involve patient in self-care and household activities.
Encourage involvement in social and recreational activities, rather than passive pastimes.
Refer to occupational therapist for aids to independence and advice regarding skills training.

DOES THE PATIENT FEEL DISSATISFIED WITH PAST LIFE OR HAVE SUBSTANTIAL REGRETS?

NO	YES
Feels fulfilled, satisfied	Feels bitter, unfulfilled

Talk about the regrets with patient.
Use a counselling approach, and guide towards a more positive assessment of the past, if possible.
Use a religious perspective where appropriate.
Understand the impact of past disappointments and be sympathetic.

DOES THE PATIENT HAVE ANY OTHER PROBLEMS TO COPE WITH?

NO	YES
Would be relatively trouble-free without pain	Loss or illness of close relative or friend Financial or domestic problems

Provide practical help with practical problems, using referrals where necessary (e.g. regarding financial difficulties).
Provide social support during periods of adjustment, and gradually encourage alternative active interests.

ARE THERE ANY OTHER POSSIBLE REASONS FOR NEGATIVE FEELINGS, E.G. DEATH ANXIETY, CONCERN ABOUT THE FUTURE, DRUGS, ALCOHOL?

Manage as appropriate.

Figure 6.2 An algorithm for the nursing management of elderly patients with pain. Reproduced from Walker, J., Akinsanya, J.A., Davis, B. & Marcer, D. (1990) The nursing management of elderly patients with pain in the community: study and recommendations. *Journal of Advanced Nursing*, **15**, 1154–1161, with kind permission of Blackwell Science Ltd.

Using routine drug rounds as the time for pain assessment does not facilitate pain assessment. At this time the nurse cannot possibly carry out a comprehensive assessment, and, as discussed in Chapter 5, the type of information collected from a patient following a request issued from a nurse who is standing at the drug trolley may be completely different from that collected while the nurse is sitting down and talking quietly with the patient.

6.4 Nursing interventions for the patient in pain

Once the cause of the patient's pain has been identified, decisions need to be made about how to ameliorate it effectively. A vast range of pharmacological and non-pharmacological interventions can be employed in the management of the different types of pain. Decisions surrounding the management of acute pain are far less complicated than those required for chronic pain. Acute pain is transient and therefore will decrease in intensity over time. The patient knows that the pain will go away eventually. In contrast, chronic pain is persistent, serves no useful purpose and can get worse over time. Complicated psycho-social and spiritual factors are much more likely to both contribute to and result from a chronic pain experience. The goals of care for acute pain are also simpler. It is often possible to aim at preventing acute pain occurring in the first place, or failing this, to aim at eradicating the pain entirely. Such a goal may be totally unrealistic with chronic pain. The goal of care with chronic pain is often to minimise pain and then to rehabilitate patients to achieve optimal functioning within the constraints imposed by their pain.

6.5 Pharmacological interventions

Administration of pain medication

In many hospitals the person with the responsibility for prescribing pain medication is the junior doctor. Junior doctors are often dependent on the advice of senior nurses about which analgesic agents to prescribe. Thus, nurses can have a huge influence on the choice and dose of analgesic agent prescribed by doctors. In addition, nurses have to make decisions about the timing of administration and the dose of analgesic agent to administer. Moreover, in some countries, suitably qualified community based nurses are now empowered to alter the timing and dosage of medications prescribed by doctors (Hunt & Wainwright, 1994). These authors suggest that in the future we will witness more and more nurses with the legal power to prescribe. It seems clear therefore that nurses should have thorough knowledge of the action of analgesic agents, their side effects, dosages and the frequency of use in different circumstances.

Choosing an appropriate analgesic

The most common pharmacological agents available for pain control and their routes of administration are summarised in Chapter 7. Here we shall consider how these drugs should be used, and the possible side effects they may cause, which usually will be managed by the nursing staff. The person prescribing an analgesic must make a number of different decisions including:

- Which analgesic agent(s) should be prescribed?
- What dose?
- Does the patient require a co-analgesic?
- Which route is appropriate?
- Is a drug delivery device necessary?

A good assessment will guide the clinician in answering many of these questions. If the patient is in pain, and there is no valid clinical reason why an analgesic agent cannot be given at the time, an analgesic should be administered immediately. The analgesic agent chosen depends on the severity of the pain. Strong opioids are required for the patient whose pain does not respond to non-opioid or weak opioid analgesics or whose pain is severe at onset. The dose of the drug should be titrated until analgesia is achieved or until side effects are unmanageable (Hammack & Loprinzi, 1994). A discussion on the management of the side effects of analgesic drugs will be provided later in this chapter. If patients do experience unmanageable side effects from an opioid analgesic, it is worth considering changing the opioid (de Stoutz *et al.*, 1995).

In general *pro re nata* (PRN: as required) dosing of analgesic agents is inappropriate for patients with chronic pain. Fixed-time-interval administration of analgesics is the more appropriate approach for chronic pain because it provides a continuous therapeutic level of drug which prevents the pain returning. Patients on a fixed-time-interval schedule should have an agent prescribed for breakthrough pain. It is often useful to have a range of doses of a particular analgesic agent included in the prescription. This gives the nurse some flexibility when deciding the most appropriate dose of analgesic agent to administer at a particular time.

The cause of the pain will ultimately dictate the choice of analgesic agent. Some pains will only be ameliorated through the use of a number of agents in combination. A discussion on the most appropriate choice of analgesic agent to choose for different pain conditions can be found in Chapter 7.

Evoking the placebo effect

In Chapter 5 the issue of using placebo pills in an unethical or fraudulent manner was addressed. The use of a placebo pill in such a way is completely different from, and should not be compared to, evoking the placebo effect for the benefit of the patient. This latter approach is often viewed by healthcare professionals in a negative light which is unfortunate since the placebo effect possesses a remarkable potency and will often act in a synergistic way with standard pharmacological treatments (Benson & Friedman, 1996). The placebo effect can be evoked by:

- a positive belief and expectation of treatment effect on the part of both patient and healthcare professional;
- enthusiastic administration of the drug;
- showing a warm, sympathetic and interested attitude towards the patient.

Thus, it could be argued that steps should be taken to foster a positive belief in the effects of the analgesic agent, and efforts should be made to demonstrate a warm, sympathetic attitude towards the patient when administering the drug. This will do the patient no harm, unlike the provision of placebo pills – on the contrary, it is likely to increase the efficacy of the prescribed treatment.

6.6 Management of the side effects of analgesic agents

A wide range of side effects are associated with analgesic agents. The development of side effects is dependent on a number of factors which include the route of administration, dosage, concurrent organ dysfunction, drug interactions and the length of time the patient has been taking the drug (Coyle *et al.*, 1995). It is important to anticipate which side effect(s) a particular patient might experience and to take steps to prevent that side effect(s) occurring.

Side effects of NSAIDs

Unfortunately, there are a number of troublesome side effects associated with non-steroidal anti-inflammatory drugs (NSAIDs) (Table 6.2). These effects can appear at any time but are more commonly associated with long-term use.

Table 6.2   Side effects of NSAIDs.

- Drug interactions
- Gastro-intestinal toxicity
- Renal and hepatic dysfunction
- Risk of bleeding
- Mask signs and symptoms of infection
- Mild salicylism
- Hypersensitivity reaction

Gastro-intestinal toxicities

Gastro-intestinal (GI) toxicities (Table 6.3) are seen quite commonly when a patient is taking NSAIDs. Patients on NSAIDs should be taught to take drugs with food or a glass of milk and never on an empty stomach. Some patients may require an antacid to prevent stomach upset. Alcohol may exacerbate stomach upset, so patients should be advised to avoid drinking it as much as possible. Minor GI disturbances may not always precede serious effects such as bleeding, perforation or ulceration; therefore the patient should be advised to report any gastro-intestinal disturbances as soon as possible.

Table 6.3   Gastro-intestinal side effects of NSAIDs.

- Dyspepsia
- Heartburn
- Gastritis
- Nausea and vomiting
- Anorexia
- Diarrhoea
- Constipation
- Flatulence
- Bloating
- Abdominal pain
- Gastric bleeding
- Ulceration
- Perforation

Risk of bleeding

Aspirin irreversibly inhibits platelet aggregation which may prolong bleeding time for several days following administration of the drug. Other NSAIDs, with the exception of nonacetylated salicylates, have a similar inhibitory effect on platelet aggregation, although this is reversible; therefore, the patient will be only at risk of bleeding for the period the drug is circulating in the blood stream. For this reason, NSAIDs are not administered to patients with thrombocytopenia or other bleeding disorders. Patients about to undergo surgery should be asked whether they have ingested aspirin in the past forty eight hours (Coyle *et al.*, 1995).

Masking indicators of infection

NSAIDs are taken for their antipyretic and anti-inflammatory effects; however, in neutropenic patients these normal effects can have catastrophic consequences. This is because NSAIDs may mask the usual signs and symptoms of infection, in particular, a raised temperature. In neutropenic patients a raised temperature may be the only sign of infection, masking this sign means that the infection may not be identified promptly, resulting in the infection progressing to septic shock, which is associated with a high mortality rate. For this reason NSAIDs are not administered normally to neutropenic patients.

Drug interactions

NSAIDs bind extensively to plasma proteins which means that they can displace or be displaced by other protein-bound drugs such as warfarin, methotrexate and digoxin. The net result of this is an increase in the therapeutic or toxic effects of either drug. In addition, NSAIDs can interact with a number of other drugs. It is important to warn the patient not to take any other medication without checking with a doctor or nurse beforehand.

Hepatic and renal dysfunction

NSAIDs can cause hepatic or renal dysfunction at any time; however, they are more likely to occur in patients who are taking these agents in the long term. Moreover, older patients and those with pre-existing renal or hepatic dysfunction are at greater risk. Patients should be advised to report any signs and symptoms which are indicative of hepatic or renal dysfunction. These would include jaundice, abdominal pain, inadequate or excessive urinary output, cystitis and haematuria. In addition, patients should be advised to avoid excessive alcohol intake. Tests of renal and hepatic function should be measured on a regular basis. This is particularly important if the patient is taking other nephrotoxic or hepatotoxic drugs.

Hypersensitivity reactions

Hypersensitivity to NSAIDs can occur within minutes of ingestion. This can take the form of a dermatological reaction which is characterised by rash, urticaria, pruritus, or dermatitis. Allergic reactions can also occur and these are characterised by hypotension, rhinitis, dyspnoea, fever and acute anaphylaxis. Patients who are sensitive to one NSAID may be also sensitive to other NSAIDs, and therefore these agents should not be administered to a patient with a past history of NSAID sensitivity. Patients should be advised to report any adverse reactions immediately.

Mild salicylism

Administration of large doses of salicylates can cause salicylism, as a result of raised serum salicylate levels (> 300 mcg/ml). It is characterised by dizziness, tinnitus, diminished hearing, nausea, vomiting, diarrhoea, mental confusion, CNS depression, headache, sweating and hyperventilation. These symptoms disappear rapidly following dose reduction.

A summary of the interventions to prevent or manage the side effects of NSAIDs is provided in Table 6.4. It should be remembered that it is inadvisable to administer NSAIDs concomitantly with each other, as this can significantly increase the risk of toxicity. Patients should be advised to note the contents of non-prescription products which they take for flu and cold, as many of them contain aspirin. NSAIDs interact with a number of other drugs which may enhance the therapeutic or toxic effects of either drug (Wilkes, *et al.*, 1994).

Table 6.4   Interventions to prevent or manage the side effects of NSAIDs.

Drug interactions
Advise patient not to take any other medication without seeking medical advice beforehand.

GI toxicity
Advise patient to take NSAID with food or milk and never on an empty stomach. Advise to report any GI toxicity as soon as possible. Avoid concurrent administration of two or more NSAIDs.

Renal and hepatic dysfunction
Asses baseline renal and hepatic function to identify patients' risk; monitor renal and hepatic function closely in patients receiving concurrent hepatotoxic or nephrotoxic drugs; teach patients to report symptoms of hepatic or renal dysfunction and to avoid excessive alcohol intake.

Risk of bleeding
With the exception of nonacetylated salycilates NSAIDs should be avoided in patients with thrombocytopenia or other bleeding disorders; teach patients to report symptoms of bleeding; avoid concurrent use of NSAIDs.

Mask signs and symptoms of infection
Avoid use of NSAIDs in neutropenic patients.

Mild salicylism
Teach patient to reduce or interrupt dose if signs of salicylism occur; assess medications for possible drug interactions.

Hypersensitivity reactions
Do not administer NSAID to patients with a history of hypersensitivity to NSAIDs; teach patients to report symptoms of hypersensitivity; provide symptomatic relief for rashes or puritus.

Side effects of opioids

Patients taking opioids may experience a great many side effects (Table 6.5). Thankfully many of these effects are rare, can be prevented, and are often only troublesome in the short term. It is unfortunate that health professionals and the general public alike hold many negative mis-

Table 6.5 Side effects of opioids.

- Respiratory depression
- Sedation
- Confusion
- Nausea and vomiting
- Dry mouth
- Constipation
- Multifocal myoclonus
- Urinary retention
- Orthostatic hypotension
- Pruritus
- Physical dependence
- Bilary spasm
- Impotence
- Amenorrhea
- Reduction in libido

conceptions about the side effects of opioids (see Chapter 5); thus, it is important that these misconceptions are corrected and the patient informed about the exact nature of the side effects of opioids and the ways in which they can be ameliorated.

Respiratory depression

Respiratory depression is the most life-threatening side effect of opioids, and most commonly occurs in opioid-naive patients with parenteral administration, particularly when pain is abruptly relieved. It is important to point out that pain is a stimulus to respiration, and therefore respiratory depression will not be manifested as a problem unless pain is controlled. Respiratory depression is often accompanied by other signs of CNS depression such as sedation. There is a time lag between drug administration and the development of respiratory depression which is dependent on the route of administration (Foley & Inturrisi, 1992). Tolerance to respiratory depression develops rapidly with long-term use of opioids.

Patients who are opioid naive or with severe lung disease and receiving parenteral opioids for the first time, should be monitored closely for respiratory depression. If it occurs, it can be reversed by IV naloxone. Naloxone should be used with great care in patients receiving opioids on a long-term basis because these patients are very sensitive to the effects of antagonist drugs and reverse analgesia can easily occur. In this situation a diluted solution of naloxone should be titrated against the patient's respiratory rate.

Sedation

Patients who wish to maintain their normal activities often find sedation to be a troublesome and unacceptable side effect of opioids. Tolerance to sedation will normally develop within a few days, although in some patients it may persist. If this occurs switching to an alternative opioid or the use of psychostimulant drugs can often reduce sedation to an acceptable level while maintaining analgesia. Some patients may see sedation as evidence of disease progression which could cause them to feel very anxious. Therefore, patients need to be warned that this is a normal side effect of opioids and that, in most instances, it will wear off in a matter of days.

A recent study demonstrated that cancer patients receiving long-term opioids with stable doses have only slightly worse scores on psychological and neurological tests relevant to driving ability when compared with cancer patients receiving no opioids (Vainio *et al.*, 1995). These authors concluded that long-term analgesic medication with stable doses of opioids does not impair driving ability. Thus, patients taking opioids in the long-term should only be asked to avoid driving if sedation is a persistent problem. This group of patients should also be advised to avoid operating machinery in this situation. Alcohol will increase sedation and should be avoided if sedation becomes a troublesome problem for the patient. Marked sedation can be an indicator of opioid-induced respiratory failure.

Nausea and vomiting

Approximately 30% of patients will experience nausea and vomiting when initially commencing on opioids (O'Brien, 1993). These symptoms are more commonly experienced by patients receiving epidural morphine. Patients are more likely to experience nausea and vomiting when they sit up or try to move around which suggests that opioids sensitise the vestibular apparatus in some way. Opioids are also thought to cause nausea and vomiting by direct stimulation of the chemoreceptor trigger zone and by their effects on gastric motility and emptying. The pain itself and constipation may be other contributory factors. Tolerance develops rapidly to this effect, although this is of little benefit to patients receiving opioids in the short term. It is important to determine the cause of nausea and vomiting before deciding what anti-emetic agent to administer. Prophylactic anti-emetic therapy is necessary for most patients in the short term, particularly those patients who have experienced opioid-induced nausea and vomiting previously. An in-depth discussion on the management of nausea and vomiting can be found in Hawthorn (1995).

Constipation

Constipation is commonly seen in patients who are taking both weak and strong opioid analgesics on a long-term basis. It is often much more difficult to treat constipation than control pain. There are numerous causes of constipation (Table 6.6) which means that some patients on opioids are at greater risk of developing constipation. For example, patients with advanced cancer often have impaired immobility, inadequate dietary intake and are taking a range of constipation causing medications. The proportion of these patients requiring laxatives rises from 65% to nearly 90% when they start taking opioids (Baines & Sykes, 1993). Laxatives should be prescribed prophylactically for patients who are at high risk of becoming constipated (Regnard, 1995). The choice of laxative is dependent on the cause of constipation; however, in opioid-induced constipation the patient normally requires a stool softener in combination with a stimulant (e.g. docusate and senna or co-danthramer). There is some evidence that senna compounds reverse opioid induced constipation by increasing intestinal motility without interfering with the analgesic effect of the opioid (Maguire *et al.*, 1990; Canty, 1994). In severe cases of constipation it may be appropriate to use metoclopramide or cisapride, although great caution needs to be exercised when using these agents in patients with gastrointestinal obstruction. There is some evidence that oral naloxone may have a role in treating opioid induced constipation that does not respond to treatment with laxatives (Coyle *et al.*, 1995; Sykes, 1996).

Other important factors to consider when deciding on which laxative to recommend is its cost and how palatable the patient finds the mixture. The dose of laxative should be titrated to maintain a patient's normal bowel movements. Rectal measures should be avoided if possible; however, if

Table 6.6   Causes of constipation.

- Inactivity
- Dehydration
- Inadequate dietary intake
- Low-fibre diet
- Obstruction of the gut
- Inability to get to the toilet
- Lack of privacy when defecating
- Paralysis
- Haemorrhoids
- Hypercalcaemia
- Hypokalaemia
- Opioids
- NSAIDs
- Drugs with anticholinergic effects
- $5HT_3$ receptor antagonists
- Tricyclic antidepressants
- Vinca alkaloids
- Aluminium antacids
- Iron

there are hard faeces in the rectum, a suppository or enema is probably necessary. If the patient is faecally impacted, a manual evacuation may be required. The patient should be sedated for this procedure.

Non-pharmacological approaches are also important in preventing or treating constipation, although opioid-induced constipation cannot usually be managed by employing non-pharmacological measures alone. Every effort should be made to provide the patient with privacy when defecating. If a patient cannot get to the toilet, a commode is preferable to a bedpan. Increased fluid and dietary fibre intake, increased exercise and regular toilet habits can help prevent constipation (Canty, 1994). Unfortunately, very ill patients may find it difficult to eat a high-fibre diet, drink enough fluid or do some exercise. In this situation good symptom control will help the patient to eat and be as active as possible (Baines & Sykes, 1993).

Dry mouth

A very unpleasant and common side effect of opioids is a dry mouth. A dry mouth can contribute to the patient developing dental caries and periodontal disease, as well as interfering with a patient's ability to eat and communicate (Holmes, 1991). There may be other factors causing a dry mouth such as reduced fluid intake, anticholinergic drugs and oral candida. Where possible these contributory factors should be treated. The most important intervention for dry mouth is regular oral hygiene. Patients should be encouraged to brush their teeth and use a mouth wash as regularly as possible. Commercial mouth washes should be avoided since they contain alcohol. Lemon and glycerine swabs should not be used since they cause damage to the dental enamel and may actually increase the dryness. Artificial salivary supplements may be beneficial. Food with a high sugar content should be avoided since it can increase the risk of dental caries.

Urinary retention

Opioids occasionally cause an increase in bladder sphincter tone which can result in urinary retention. This is most commonly seen with the administration of spinal opioids and in patients with prostatism or urethral stricture. Tolerance to this effect develops rapidly; however, in some instances catheterisation may be required. Patients should be asked to report any difficulty with urination.

Confusion

Mild cognitive impairment can result when the patient begins taking opioids, but it usually resolves within a few days. In patients who already have some degree of confusion, opioids can exacerbate the condition. Therefore, these patients need to be monitored closely for any change in their cognitive status.

Pruritus

Pruritus occurs most commonly after epidural and spinal administration of opioids and is frequently localised to the face. Patients should be warned of this side effect; and if the itching proves to be troublesome, antihistamines may be beneficial in some patients.

Multifocal myoclonus

High doses of opioids can cause myoclonus which are shock-like, involuntary muscular contractions. It is seen most commonly following the repeated administration of large doses of pethedine (>250 mg per day) (Foley & Inturrisi, 1992) or in the patient with advanced cancer in the last 48 hours of life (O'Brien, 1993). Interventions for this effect include switching to a different opioid or using anxiolytics to suppress myoclonic jerks. Patients need to be reassured that this is a normal, although uncommon, side effect. This is a particularly difficult symptom for families to witness when a loved one is dying. They also need to be reassured that this effect is normal and that the anxiolytic agents will ameliorate any distress the patient may be experiencing.

Orthostatic hypotension

Orthostatic hypotension due to vasodilatation can occur following rapid IV administration of opioids leaving the patient feeling quite faint. Care should be taken when administering IV opioids, and patients should be advised to stay lying down for a short period of time following the injection.

Suppression of cough reflex

An active cough reflex reduces the risk of chest infection in postoperative patients and since opioids can suppress the cough reflex, some patients to whom these agents are administered are at greater risk of developing a chest infection. However, the risk of suppressing the cough reflex must be weighed against the risk of the patient being unable to breathe deeply or cough because of fear of aggravating pain, since this is more likely to result in pulmonary complications. The answer is to carefully titrate the opioid against the patient's pain. This should significantly reduce the risk of suppressing the cough reflex.

Sexual dysfunction

Some men and women will experience sexual dysfunction and a reduction in libido associated with prolonged use of opioids (Wilkes *et al.*, 1994). Suppression of gonadotrophins may be responsible for these effects. The patient needs to be warned that this is a potential side effect. If the patient experiences major psychological difficulties from this effect, referral for psycho-sexual counselling is warranted.

Physical dependence

Physical dependence may occur with long-term use of opioids and refers to the precipatation of withdrawal symptoms when an opioid is stopped abruptly or if an opioid antagonist is administered. Withdrawal symptoms may be seen as soon as 2 to 3 days after repeated opioid administration. This phenomenon should not be confused with addiction or psychological dependence (see Chapter 5). Withdrawal symptoms can be prevented by making sure that the opioid is not stopped suddenly and by avoiding the use of opioid agonist-antagonist drugs. Patients should be warned that this is a potential problem and encouraged to follow their 'round the clock' pain relief regimen. If for any reason patients are unable to take their medications orally, opioids should be administered by some other route. Regardless of which route is chosen, it is important to ensure that an equianalgesic dose of opioid is administered. A summary of the interventions required to prevent or manage the side effects of opioids is provided in Table 6.7.

6.7 Non-pharmacological interventions

Patient and family education

There is a growing acceptance amongst healthcare professionals throughout the world that patients have the right to be fully informed about their disease and treatment (World Health Organisation, 1994) and that many would welcome the opportunity to become more active participants in decisions about their own care. Active participation in care has the potential to improve physical and psychological well-being, facilitate adaptation to illness and enable patients to cope more effectively with their illness experience. A prerequisite for patient participation in decision making is that they are given enough information about their disease and treatment and that they fully understand this information. Patient education and information giving will help achieve this goal.

Myths and misconceptions about pain and its treatments are common in many cultures (see Chapter 5). Such myths and misconception can result in patients:

Table 6.7 Interventions to prevent or manage the side effects of opioids.

Nausea and vomiting
Administer anti-emetic – if due to stimulation of the CTZ, try haloperidol or
prochlorperazine; if gastric statis, try metoclopramide, domperidone or cisapride;
utilise non-pharmacological interventions.

Constipation
Give prophylactic stool softener in combination with bowel stimulant; increase
fluid intake, fibre in diet and exercise if possible; establish a regular toilet habit;
consider prokinetic agents e.g. metoclopramide.

Respiratory depression
Monitor respiratory rate, particularly in opioid-naive patients and with IV opioids;
administer naloxone if respiratory depression occurs; tolerance develops rapidly.

Sedation
Try to persist for a few days; reduce dose then increase gradually if sedation
problematic; if persistent change opioid or use psychostimulant; consider adjuvant
analgesic e.g. NSAID to reduce opioid dose; eliminate any non-essential CNS
depressant medication.

Dry mouth
Treat any contributory causes; regular oral hygiene; try artificial salivary stimulants;
avoid food with high sugar content.

Multifocal myoclonus
Warn patient of potential effects; change opioid or use anxiolytic.

Confusion
Opioids may exacerbate any pre-existing confusion. Vulnerable patients should
therefore be monitored closely; changing opioids may be useful.

Orthostatic hypotension
Monitor BP following rapid IV dosing; ask patient to remain lying down for 15
minutes following rapid IV injection.

Suppression of cough reflex
Monitor patients who may be susceptible to chest infection. Titrate opioid dose
carefully to avoid suppression of the reflex.

Sexual dysfunction
Warn patients of potential side effects; consider referring for psycho-sexual
counselling if patient having psychological difficulties.

Puritus
Use antihistamines if patient finds side effects troublesome.

Physical dependence
Do not discontinue opioid suddenly.

Urinary retention
Ask patient to report any problem with urination; catheterise if necessary.

- refusing to either take analgesics;
- refusing to have the dose of analgesics increased.

Patients may also become very frightened and anxious about the future. This may result in an increase in pain perception. Information giving and patient education can alleviate anxiety by providing a realistic account of what will happen to the patient and by dispelling any myths and misconceptions a patient might hold. These benefits have been demonstrated in a number of studies. For example, Hayward (1975) found that providing patients with detailed procedural information led to a reduction in postoperative pain and anxiety. Similarly, Davis (1984) found that when patients were given pre-operative information about what to expect postoperatively and advice on coping with post-operative complications they experienced less pain. In patients with chronic pain, the provision of information about the cause and likely progress of a painful condition is thought to facilitate coping (Marcer *et al.*, 1990). In addition, it has been shown that patients who receive drug-related education have improved pain relief, better compliance with pain medication regimens, and less concerns about taking opioids than patients who have not received such education (Rimer *et al.*, 1987).

Forewarning patients about the possibility of experiencing pain can help them feel that it is legitimate to express any discomfort (Bourbonnais, 1981). Moreover, forewarning patients about the possibility of experiencing pain in an unexpected site, such as in the shoulder following a cholecystectomy, can prevent the patient becoming alarmed. Coaching patients to report their pain in a way that is understood by healthcare professionals may reduce the discrepancy between patients' self-reports and nurses' assessment of pain (Wilkie *et al.*, 1995).

An important first step in patient education is establishing what patients want to know, not what the nurse thinks they need to know. Some people will require extensive information about their illness, others want to know very little. Regardless of the amount of information a patient requires, it should be delivered in a simple and straightforward manner. Medical jargon should be avoided as much as possible. It is very hard for people to remember a large amount of information, especially if they feel anxious. People have a tendency to remember best the instructions given at the beginning of an interaction, a phenomenon referred to as the 'primacy effect' (Ley, 1972). It is therefore prudent to provide the patient with small amounts of information at one time and to check out the level of understanding as the session progresses. Oral information should be supplemented with written materials and audio-visual materials if they are available locally. In situations where patients have responsibility for the administration of their own medication, the provision of a written plan of the dosage and timing of their medication and a pill box may help facilitate compliance with the prescribed treatment.

Under a recent European Union (EU) law all drugs sold by pharmacies in EU Member States must be accompanied by an information sheet about the drug. Patients may require some help in deciphering the information contained in these leaflets.

Families also have a need for education, particularly if they are to be involved in the patient's care at home. Family members often have to decide what pain medication to give, how much to give and when to give it (Ferrell *et al.*, 1991). Moreover, they have to provide physical, social and psychological support for the patient. A family member's response to expressions of pain can ameliorate a pain problem, or alternatively can exacerbate it and culture it into chronicity (Snelling, 1994). Families, as with patients, possess a limited knowledge about pain and its management and often harbour myths and misconceptions about pain and use of opioids. Family education should be aimed at equipping family members with knowledge about the administration of drugs and preventing side effects; with dispelling myths and misconceptions and how to respond effectively to the patient's expressions of pain.

It should be remembered that patient and family education is an ongoing process, not a one-off event. There must be time for 'restating, clarifying and re-enforcing information as a person's capacity, desire and readiness for learning fluctuate.' (Grahn & Johnson, 1990.)

Positioning

Careful positioning has an important contribution to make to the management of pain (Wilkie *et al.*, 1989). Nurses should encourage patients to use a favoured position when they are hospitalised, and efforts should be made to ensure that they are not moved unless it is necessary. Pillows or other supports should be provided to help maintain a favoured position (Wilkie *et al.*, 1989). The bedside locker, bell and other control devices should be placed in an easily accessible position so that patients do not need to stretch too far, which may exacerbate their pain. Clearly, the benefits of maintaining a patient in one position has to be weighed against the risks inherent in excessive immobilisation or restrictive positioning which include chest infection, deep venous thrombosis and decubitus ulcer formation. If patients are adopting a potentially harmful position, they should be encouraged to use other, less harmful, positions.

Maintaining a balance between activity and rest

Fatigue can be a significant problem for hospitalised patients, and the maintenance of a balance between activity and rest is an important intervention to ameliorate this problem. Rest can be facilitated through the provision of appropriate lighting, temperature, ventilation and noise levels (Fordham & Dunn, 1994), although it must be acknowledged that it is sometimes extremely difficult to control these factors in an acute hospital setting. Rest can also be facilitated through some thoughtful planning about when procedures and tests should be carried out and the use of complementary interventions such as relaxation therapy and aromatherapy (see Chapter 8 for a more complete discussion on complementary interventions).

Many patients with chronic pain are in a very poor physical state as a result of sleep deprivation with some patients complaining of being eternally 'jet-lagged' (Meinhart & McMaffrey, 1983). Sleep deprivation can result in loss of concentration and less energy to cope with the pain experience. Inactivity as a result of the pain can exacerbate the problem. Some patients will require a bedtime sedative. Rankin (1982) suggests that merely having the option of a bedtime sedative helps some patients to sleep better. Patients with low back pain should avoid sleeping in a prone position, and the use of a firm mattress or a bedboard is recommended (Jacobs, 1985).

Environment

Some hospital environments do little to facilitate a person to achieve and maintain a sense of privacy. According to Wainwright (1985) lack of privacy can increase anxiety and make patients feel that they have lost their independence and control over a situation. This in turn can increase pain perception. Lack of privacy may also inhibit a person's expression of pain and act as a barrier to communication (Fagerhaugh & Strauss, 1977). A pleasant physical environment can be created by providing the patient with access to a private space and control over lighting, temperature and ventilation. Moreover, distraction can be facilitated by assigning a patient to a room with a working television set or radio and through the provision of flexible visiting hours. However, the benefits of distraction from visitors should be weighed against the patient's need for rest. Although it may be difficult to make any major changes to the environment in a hospital setting, it seems clear that careful consideration needs to be given as to how a hospital environment can be used more creatively to facilitate the patient to maintain as much privacy, independence and control as possible (Wainwright, 1985).

Interventions for patients with acute pain

Acute pain is most commonly managed within a hospital setting. This can pose problems in terms of achieving good continuity of care and therefore, good pain control. Strategies to achieve optimal control of acute pain include the establishment of an acute pain service and the provision of protocols for the management of acute pain (Royal College of Surgeons and College of Anaesthetists, 1990; Gould *et al.*, 1992; Mackintosh & Bowles, 1997). The contribution of non-pharmacological interventions to the management of acute pain should not be overlooked.

Interventions for women in labour

Acute pain is an integral component of giving birth, the memory of which will remain with a woman for the rest of her life. The pain of childbirth differs from other acute pains in terms of its meaning, in that it occurs as a result of natural events and because its severity and length is more unpredictable (Cianciolo Livingstone, 1985; Moore, 1997). The woman's attitude towards childbirth will very much influence her choice of pain relief strategy. Some women wish to experience a completely natural childbirth without any medical intervention, others prefer to have a pain-free labour and therefore, need to have a range of pharmacological interventions available to them. Both the 'natural' and 'pain-free' approaches can result in a rewarding emotional experience; however, there can be also disadvantages associated with both approaches (Moore, 1997). For example, some women have expressed dissatisfaction with a 'pain-free' birth since they were left with no sense of achievement; other women would find the pain of a 'natural' childbirth too much to bear and be left physically and emotionally exhausted from the experience. The midwife has an important role to play in determining each woman's pain control needs during labour and ensuring that these needs are met.

A number of non-pharmacological approaches have been used with various degrees of success to control labour pain including:

- relaxation (Bamfield, 1997);
- changing the maternal position (Simkins, 1989; Melzack *et al.*, 1991);
- immersion in water (Alderdice & Marchant, 1997);
- massage (Moore & Holden, 1997);
- aromatherapy (Mason, 1995; Stevensen, 1995);
- music (Cianciolo Livingston, 1985);
- acupuncture (Moore & Holden, 1997);
- hypnosis (Rankin-Box, 1995);
- transcutaneous electrical nerve stimulation (TENS) (Davies, 1997);
- biofeedback (Duchene, 1989).

It is beyond the scope of this book to discuss the use of the above mentioned interventions in depth; however, a discussion on some of the cognitive-behavioural strategies and TENS can be found in Chapter 8. Furthermore, an excellent discussion on labour pain and its management can be found in the book edited by Moore (1997).

Intervention for patients with chronic pain

The largest group of patients with chronic pain are those with chronic benign pain who are medically stable and do not require aggressive medical interventions. This group of patients poses a huge challenge for healthcare professionals, and many cases are poorly managed. Life with chronic pain can result in the patient developing numerous behavioural and emotional problems, many of which are maladaptive and include ineffective coping strategies, over-reliance on pain relief medication, disruption in personal relationships, sexual problems, feelings of hopelessness and loss of control. Given the complexity and multi-dimensionality of the chronic benign pain experience, it is important that it is viewed as a completely different entity to acute pain and that assessment and management strategies reflect this difference (Seers & Friedli 1996).

A key difference between benign chronic pain and acute pain is that palliation of symptoms may actually have a deleterious effect on chronic benign pain. According to Slater and Good (1991) patients' level of function will not automatically improve once their symptoms have been ameliorated – the converse is generally true. These authors suggest that improvements in pain perception more often follows increases in functional capacity. Thus, the primary focus of treatment should be rehabilitation. Gaskin *et al.* (1992) point out that the focusing of cognitive treatment on specific problems such as anger or anxiety is probably more effective for the individual chronic pain patient than a generic pain management programme. For this reason the rehabilitation programme should be individualised and should combine patient and family education, physical reconditioning and behaviour management.

Pains which lack a well-defined physical cause, as is the case with many of the chronic benign pains, are sometimes categorised as being psychogenic in nature (Bendelow & Williams, 1995). This can have disasterous consequences for patients with chronic benign pain since it often results in their pain not being believed by health professionals. This belief is transmitted very easily to family members and the patient can end up being labelled as 'a neurotic', 'a malingerer' or as having a pain that is 'all in the head'. This can be a source of considerable frustration and upset for patients. Those with chronic benign pain possess a strong need to have their pain acknowledged and legitimised by both health professionals and family members (Reid *et al.*, 1991; Rose, 1994; Seers & Friedli, 1996). Therefore, believing the patient's pain is a fundamental component of a pain rehabilitation programme.

Behaviour management

A behaviour management programme is pivotal to rehabilitating the patient with chronic pain. Such a programme seeks to reinforce healthy behaviours and to discourage those that maintain pain, dysfunction and disability. A structured plan of action should be drawn up where specific daily goals are set. All agreed activities such as taking medication or exercise should be undertaken according to a schedule. This will help the patient to develop better ways to ameliorate pain and maintain function. A pivotal element of this programme is for both the treatment team and family members to ignore maladaptive behaviours and to reward adaptive behaviours. This is thought to help break the cycle of dysfunction and disability which can be so destructive. Continuous feedback on progress towards achieving goals should be provided.

Patients with chronic pain may present with numerous problems associated with taking their pain medication. Many have stockpiled tablets over the years and end up taking their medications in ineffective and harmful combinations, which results in various side effects. Furthermore, some patients abuse or become overly reliant on their pain medication. This may actually increase or perpetuate pain through rebound effects. Patients may enter a rehabilitation programme requiring detoxification. There can be significant problems associated with withdrawal from pain medication and therefore, a structured, medically supervised programme is required. Sudden withdrawal of opioids should be avoided. Following the process of detoxification, new medication should be introduced on a strict time schedule within the context of a behavioural management programme. An important aspect of such a programme is to help patients believe that they are in control of their medication use. Eventually, some patients will be able to discontinue their medication completely.

A structured programme of physical exercises should be developed as part of the behaviour management programme. Exercise can:

- decrease muscle strain;
- increase mobility;
- produce competing stimuli for pain impulses;
- conserve energy;
- reduce fatigue (Vandenbosch, 1985).

Learning to pace activities is important. Embarking on an intensive exercise programme or an ambitious project following months or even years of inactivity is not a good idea. A schedule of regular activity followed by rest is more prudent. When planning a schedule, the level of exercise or activity that each patient is encouraged to undertake should be determined by structural and functional limitations. With most patients it will be important to start slowly, with exercises requiring very low levels of effort. If this proves successful, patients will gain confidence and be more willing to increase their level of activity. Progress should be charted to demonstrate to the patient that an increase in functional capacity is possible despite the presence of pain and can actually help decrease their pain in the long term. Some patients will need to be convinced that an increase in pain in the short term will be worth it in the long term. An increase in functional capacity will facilitate some patients to re-establish a social life and in some situations, find new employment.

The range of activities undertaken by some patients may be restricted for some very simple reasons. Often an assessment of a patient's home by an occupational therapist, where available, or a community nurse can result in modifications which can greatly simplify activities and encourage the patient to become more active.

Patients with chronic pain often experience nutritional problems. There are a number of possible reasons for this including:

- difficulty in preparing well-balanced meals due to pain;
- inactivity;
- depression;
- financial difficulties;
- gastrointestinal side effects of pain medication.

An adequate, well-balanced diet helps to maintain optimal energy levels, which in turn contributes to the patient's willingness to undertake various activities. It is important to determine the cause of any nutritional problem before deciding the most appropriate interventions. For one patient, the organisation of a meals-on-wheels service may be the answer, for another, it may be changing pain medication or advice on how to prevent gastro-intestinal side effects.

It is highly probable that patients with chronic pain who were pre-viously employed in jobs which required heavy labour will be unable to return to work and will therefore be living on some form of disability benefit. An increase in functional capacity may help the patient to feel more able to undertake job retraining. New employment will help patients overcome some of the financial difficulties which often plague their lives. It may also help the patient maintain a sense of meaning and purpose in life.

Many of the supportive therapies (Chapter 8), particularly cognitive techniques, have an important role in helping patients with chronic pain gain some control over their pain. Often these techniques help patients to look at their pain in a different way and come to accept that pain is a part of their life; however, it does not need to dominate that life. This will allow patients to establish a sense of control over their pain, which in turn may affect their perceptions of pain and how they respond to their pain (Bates *et al.*, 1993).

Relationships within families, particularly between partners, can be badly affected by a chronic pain experience. Moreover, a spouse's solici-tous response to a patient's pain behaviours may cause the patient to experience greater physical dysfunction and an increase in pain behaviours (Romano *et al.*, 1995). Therefore it is important that spouses and other family members are included in the rehabilitation programme.

Some family members may need support in their own right. A change in the status of a married couple's relationship, often from one of equality to one where the patient becomes dependent, can lead to conflict within the marriage. This may place a huge burden on both individuals and can lead to sexual difficulties or separation. Marital and sexual counselling may be required to help overcome these personal conflicts.

Sternbach (1987) has provided a set of guiding principles for patients on how they might best achieve mastery over their pain (Table 6.8). This table provides a useful summary of the advice patients should be given on completion of their behavioural management programme.

Table 6.8 Sternbach's principles for mastering chronic pain.

- Accept that you have chronic pain.
- Set specific goals for work, hobbies and social activities and then work towards these goals.
- Let yourself get angry at your pain if it seems to be getting the best of you.
- Take your pain killers on a strict time schedule, and then taper off until you are no longer taking any.
- Get into the best physical shape possible, and keep fit.
- Learn how to relax, and practice relaxation techniques regularly.
- Keep busy but learn to pace your activities.
- Encourage your family and friends to support your healthy behaviours, not your invalidism.
- Be open and reasonable with your doctors.
- Remain hopeful.

Source: Sternbach (1987).

The management of chronic pain normally takes place in a community setting. This means that all the community resources available need to be mobilised. Hospital-based nurses should plan the patient's discharge carefully and ensure that resources are in place before the patient returns home. There is often a breakdown in communication between different care settings. This is sometimes caused by the fact that no one professional co-ordinates the situation. If chronic pain is to be managed effectively, a seamless service should be provided. One of the health professionals involved in a patient's care should be nominated as co-ordinator and take charge of communications between all those services involved. Such proactive planning may help prevent the patient 'falling between two stools' and ensure the provision of an optimal rehabilitation service.

Interventions for patients with advanced cancer

Life with advanced cancer can be incredibly burdensome for the patient. It is a time of enormous loss – loss of physical strength and bodily function, loss of role both within the family and wider community and loss of life. It is also a time when feelings of anxiety, anger, fear, loneliness and depression predominate. Since all of these emotions can increase pain perception, it is not surprising that the use of non-pharmacological interventions forms an integral and important component of the management of cancer pain. Good communication is the most important of these interventions since it facilitates patients to explore their frustrations, anxieties and fears and to find some meaning in their present life situation. Other interventions to facilitate the patient's search for meaning in cancer pain have been outlined by Ferrell and Dean (1995) and include:

- provide aggressive pharmacological pain management to achieve optimum pain relief;
- include non-pharmacological interventions that enhance a sense of control;
- assist patients in verbalising and understanding the cause of their pain, clarify physiological causes of pain;
- explore with patients and family members their images of pain including metaphors, visions;
- overcome barriers to optimum use of analgesic, such as fear of addiction;
- distinguish the feelings or meaning attributed to pain from those beliefs about death;
- empower patients to assume an active role in pain assessment and management;
- explore the losses associated with the illness and pain;
- facilitate discussion between patients and family caregivers to acquire a shared meaning of pain;
- encourage comparison of the patient's pain to that experienced by others;
- identify limits to pain that patients perceive to be necessary or deserved;
- facilitate spiritual interventions including spiritual counselling, rituals, prayer;
- explore pain as a sign of hopelessness and foster altered hope consistent with advancing disease.

It takes time and energy on the part of both the patient and nurse to engage actively in a process which will elucidate the many factors contributing to the patient's perception of pain. Saunders (1988) points out that sometimes patients are too ill to engage in this process and staff may be too busy. She suggests that we often have to accept the reality of this situation; however, we can persevere with the practical. For example, the way nursing care is given, the way we take time to question a patient about a symptom or the way we accept the patient's and family's anger may go some way towards ameliorating the patient's pain. Some patients with advanced cancer will have pain which will not respond to appropriate pharmacological and non-pharmacological interventions. This may be because the pain has a deep emotional component, and more sophisticated psychological interventions are required in order for patients to acknowledge and give expression to the emotional component of their pain (Kearney, 1992; 1996). These psychological interventions should only be provided by professionals who have undergone specific training in this area.

Cancer pain can be reduced by a number of pain control behaviours including positioning, distraction and pressure manipulation. Over a lifetime of experiencing different types of pain, patients will have discovered a range of idiosyncratic pain relieving remedies. Some patients may be inhibited about using these remedies whilst hospitalised because they fear being ridiculed by staff, even though they probably use them all of the time at home (Copp, 1974; Wilkie *et al.*, 1989). Thus, the onus is on the nurse to determine which pain control behaviours are helpful for the patient and then to facilitate the patient to use these behaviours as frequently as necessary. This should enhance the patient's sense of control. Poor positioning can exacerbate pain, therefore helping the bed-bound and weak patient to maintain a comfortable position with pillows and other supports and minimising the amount of times they have to move are important interventions. The use of distraction and other cognitive-behavioural techniques also have an important role to play in ameliorating cancer pain. In addition, the provision of basic nursing interventions can make a huge difference to a patient's level of comfort. For example, good oral care can make the patient's dry mouth feel more comfortable, enable them to eat food and facilitates communication.

The physical environment can effect a patient's mood, which in turn can increase pain perception. When hospitalised, some patients express a desire to touch their own possessions and to walk around in a familiar environment. Therefore, the provision of a pleasant and familiar environment can provide significant comfort for the patient. In a hospital or hospice setting such an environment can be created by encouraging the patient to bring in favourite items such as pillows, plants, towels, books, pictures or photographs from home.

6.8 Monitoring the patient

The patient's pain will change over time regardless of whether it is acute or chronic in nature. This means that the progress of a patient's pain should be monitored on a regular basis to determine whether interventions have worked or whether the condition has resolved. Unfortunately, there are no clear guidelines as to how frequently the various different types of pain should be monitored; moreover, with more chronic forms of pain the optimal timing of assessment may be difficult to define (Deschampes *et al.*, 1988). Chronic pain should be re-assessed regularly enough to cover sufficiently the range of activities the patient carries out every day, whereas acute pain demands more frequent re-assessment in the short term, with the frequency of assessment reduced as the painful condition improves.

The use of measurement tools is an important means of assessing whether or not the interventions have been effective. It should be remembered that the same measurement tool should be used on each occasion the pain(s) is monitored.

When monitoring the patient's pain there are a number of related issues that need to be considered. First, remember that some patients do not want to be reminded of their pain, particularly when they are using purposeful distraction. Give careful consideration to the frequency of monitoring pain in this group of patients. It is often easy to assume that they are not in pain because they are not exhibiting 'normal' pain expression behaviours (see Chapter 5). In the post-operative setting the patient's pain description may indicate complications, and therefore your index of suspicion should be increased if the pain descriptions change dramatically. Finally, be aware of a person's typical behaviour when in pain – a stoic patient complaining of pain is significant, as is a previously demonstrative patient becoming silent and withdrawn (Copp, 1974).

6.9 Considerations in children

There are many commonalties between the management of pain in children and adults; nevertheless, some differences do exist and deserve discussion in a book of this nature. As with adults, accurate assessment of a child's pain is central to effective management. In a child, the approach to assessment is heavily dependent on the age and development stage of the child. Many of the self-report scales used for adults can be used for most children aged seven or over (Van Keuren & Eland, 1997). A number of picture and colour scales have been developed for children aged three to seven which have shown good reliability and validity (Van Keuren & Eland, 1997). In pre-verbal and non-verbal children, observation for behavioural expressions of pain is a central component of assessment (Shandor Miles & Neelon, 1989). Mills (1989) has identified five types of behaviours associated with acute pain in infants and toddlers which include:

- specific motor movements (e.g. kicking, jerking, pulling away, clenching fists, arching, etc.);
- vocalisations and verbalisations (e.g. crying, calling for parents, expressing pain, telling what hurts, etc.);
- change in facial expression (e.g. grimacing, frowning, pouting, etc.);

- changes in interactions with parents and care-givers (e.g. clinging, avoiding eye contact, expressing anger and aggression, loss of interest in play);
- attempts at self-consolation (e.g. lying still, seeking escape, self-biting, seeking comfort, biting a towel, etc.).

These behaviours vary considerably according to the child's age and pain intensity. Parents are an important source of information about how their child normally copes with and expresses pain. Unfortunately, the parents' contribution is often overlooked and sometimes not believed (Hamers *et al.*, 1996).

Children are able to report pain from an early age. Pain words will appear early in a child's vocabulary, with the number and complexity of words used increasing with age (Tesler *et al.*, 1989). The pain descriptors children use can provide valuable information about the quality of their pain, and measurement tools have been developed based on such descriptors (Tesler *et al.*, 1989; Wilkie *et al.*, 1990; Abu-Saad *et al.*, 1994). It is important to be aware of and to document the particular set of words an individual child uses to describe pain.

A child's self-report of and behavioural responses to pain will be influenced by a number of factors including:

- stress associated with hospitalisation causing fear, anxiety and loss of control;
- fear of further painful procedures such as having an injection;
- a wish to protect parents;
- a desire to please others;
- a desire to get home sooner;
- extreme illness and weakness;
- depression and apathy.

Close attention needs to be paid to these extraneous factors when assessing pain; otherwise, mistakes will be made which will result in the child experiencing unnecessary pain. Remember a lack of pain expression does not mean lack of pain. In the case of uncertainty about the existance of the child's pain, the US Agency for Health Care Policy and Research (1992) recommend that an analgesic drug be used for diagnostic purposes.

Procedures involving needles are considered painful by children. Efforts should be made to minimise the discomfort associated with procedures such as venepunctures and bone marrow aspirates. The child and family need to be prepared adequately for the procedure, and parents should be allowed stay with the child during the procedure. The use of non-pharmacological methods such as distraction, guided imagery, relaxation, bubble blowing and the application of ice may also help to reduce procedure related pain (Broome *et al.*, 1993; Hockenberry-Eaton & Sigler-Price, 1994). The strategy chosen should be appropriate for the child's level of development. Furthermore, the application of a local anaesthetic cream, such as EMLA, two hours before the start of a painful procedure is an important pharmacological intervention (Hester *et al.*, 1992). If the child is to have repeated painful procedures, it is prudent to ensure that the first one is as painless as possible in order to minimise anticipatory anxiety before subsequent procedures.

6.10 Considerations in elderly patients

The management of pain in the elderly presents a number of challenges for healthcare professionals. Elderly people are more likely than their younger counterparts to experience both acute and chronic pain (Closs, 1996). This is particularly so with institutionalised elderly (Ferrell *et al.*, 1990). Age-related factors may complicate both the assessment and management of pain in elderly patients. Failing sight and hearing, cognitive impairment, confusion and dementia create communication difficulties and therefore, pose significant barriers to pain assessment, especially in the use of measurement tools. Moreover, elderly patients are often reluctant to report their pain for fear of being a nuisance or simply because they believe that nothing can be done for their pain (Yates *et al.*, 1995).

Polypharmacy as a result of multiple medical conditions is a significant problem in elderly patients. Drug pharmacokinetics can be altered as a result of age-related changes in renal and hepatic function. These factors place the patient at greater risk of developing drug interactions and side effects (Jacox *et al.*, 1994). The dose of analgesic agent may need to be modified to prevent problems occurring. Some side effects occur more frequently in elderly patients. For example, some analgesics will have anti-cholinergic or sedative action which may cause or exacerbate sedation and confusion in elderly patients. Orthostatic hypotension which occurs following the administration of many of the medications used in pain management will increase the patient's risk of falling and fractures. Falls and fractures can have devastating consequences for the elderly person because they cause more pain, immobility and reduce independence.

A number of the common misconceptions about pain are prevalent amongst the elderly. This may contribute to the problem of non-compliance with treatment. Non-compliance may also be caused by communication difficulties, poor information giving on the part of the healthcare professional, complicated drug regimens, poor social support, poor memory, inadequate use of reminders and confusion. Clearly, compliance with treatment will be increased if misconceptions are dispelled, and special efforts made to avoid or overcome the other contributory factors.

The guidelines developed by Walker *et al.* (1990) (see Figure 6.2) outline a comprehensive approach to the nursing management of elderly patients with pain. Although developed for the management of pain in a community setting, it offers a useful guide for the care of hospitalised elderly patients with pain.

Summary of Chapter 6

- A good assessment is the cornerstone in the successful management of any distressing symptom since it enables healthcare
  professionals to make decisions about which interventions are
  appropriate for each particular patient.
- Pain is a multi-dimensional phenomenon, and efforts should be
  made to establish the many factors which may be contributing to a
  patient's pain experience. Much of this information will not be
  immediately apparant or available, which highlights the fact that
  assessment is not just a one-off event.
- Since the patient's own expression of pain is the 'gold standard' in
  assessment, effective communication is the most important
  assessment strategy.
- Measurement tools provide objective data about the patient's pain
  which is difficult for health professionals to ignore.
- The nurse has a pivitol role to play in determining the dose, timing
  and route of administration of a particular analgesic agent.
- The development of side effects is dependent on a number of
  factors including the route of administration, concurrent organ
  dysfunction, drug interactions and the length of time the patient
  has been taking the drug. Side effects need to be anticipated and
  measures put in place to prevent their occurrence.
- Evoking the placebo effect may benefit the patient since it can act
  in a synergistic way with the prescribed analgesic agents.
- Encouraging patients to participate actively in care may improve
  their physical and psychological well-being and facilitate adaptation to illness.
- Families have a need for education, particularly if they are directly
  involved in caring for the patient.
- Acute pain is an integral component of giving birth, and a
  woman's attitude towards childbirth will have a strong influence
  on her choice of pain relief strategy.
- Chronic benign pain is often managed poorly and poses an
  enormous challenge for healthcare professionals. A behaviour
  management programme is pivotal to rehabilitating the patient
  with this type of pain.
- Life with advanced cancer can place enormous burdens on the
  patient, and special efforts are required to facilitate the patient to
  find meaning in this experience.
- Since the patient's pain will change over time, it is important that it
  is monitored on a sufficiently regular basis.
- The management of pain in both children and the elderly require
  special consideration.

Chapter 7

Treatment of Pain: Pharmacological and Surgical Techniques

As the causes of pain are multifactorial, there are of necessity a variety of approaches to treating pain. Choosing an appropriate treatment is a complex clinical decision which will depend on the cause of the pain, the underlying disease(s) and the patient's general health. It must also be remembered that there may be an emotional, psychological or spiritual component to the pain, and these will need to be encompassed within the treatment. Thus, pain must be approached in an holistic manner, considering the whole patient and not just one aspect of his condition. Pain is a constantly changing phenomenon, and a crucial component of effective pain management is to incorporate a review and re-evaluation procedure. This is discussed further in Chapter 6.

This chapter will cover the pharmacological interventions and surgical techniques for pain control; non-invasive and complementary techniques are covered in Chapter 8.

There are several different types of pharmacological agents available for pain relief. In this chapter they are divided into:

- systemic analgesic drugs – systemic drugs which are designed to relieve pain directly;
- adjuvant drugs which 'help' or 'assist' the primary analgesic drug. They may not have pain as their primary indication;
- topical anaesthetics and analgesics – drugs which are rubbed on to a painful area or used prophylactically to prevent pain before, for example, an injection;
- drugs for specific conditions – those which relieve the pain of certain conditions such as nitroglycerines for angina.

7.1 Systemic analgesic drugs

A commonly used system for classifying analgesic drugs separates them into three groups of increasing analgesic properties: non-opioid drugs, weak opioids and strong opioids. These drugs may be administered alone or supplemented with adjuvant medication. A widely accepted scheme for their use is the three-step analgesic ladder devised by the World Health

Organisation (WHO, 1990). Although directed primarily at those with cancer pain this scheme will be covered in detail as the general principles apply to all patients requiring potent systemic analgesics.

7.2 The WHO analgesic ladder

The WHO ladder is represented in Figure 7.1. Using this ladder individual treatment is devised for each patient by starting at the bottom of the ladder and progressing upwards until the pain is controlled. Obviously there is scope for increasing pain control within a single 'step' by increasing doses of medication or by administering more than one drug. Dose titration of opioids is considered in greater detail below.

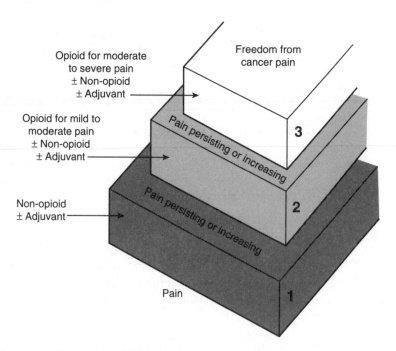

Figure 7.1 The WHO analgesic ladder. Reproduced from *Cancer Pain Relief*, 2nd edn, by kind permission of WHO, Geneva.

Step 1: Non-opioid drugs are the first line of analgesia. They usually control mild pain and where necessary may be supplemented with adjuvant drugs. Non-opioids are often underestimated as analgesics, and there is a tendency to forget how useful they can be as the patient progresses up the ladder.

Step 2: If the regimen employed in Step 1 fails to control pain, or the patient reports increasing pain, then the second line of analgesic therapy is to move to a weak opioid. The weak opioid may be given with the non-opioid or used to completely replace the non-opioid drug. Again, adjuvant drugs may be added as necessary.

Step 3: Continuing pain demands the use of a strong opioid. There is scope for greater pain control by using more potent routes of administration.

These factors are considered in detail below. Strong opioids can also be given in conjunction with adjuvant drugs or non-opioid analgesics. Some drugs such as aspirin or some NSAIDs have a 'morphine sparing effect' and thus allow the same pain relief to be achieved with a lower dose of opioid. Remember it is possible to move down the ladder, as well as up, as the patient's condition improves.

7.3 Non-opioid analgesics

The non-opioid analgesics are: acetaminophen (paracetamol), nefopam, the non-steroidal anti-inflammatory analgesics (NSAIDs).

There are many differences between non-opioid and opioid drugs. One of the most important features to remember is that non-opioids have a 'ceiling' or limit to their analgesic efficacy. That is, once the maximum dose has been reached further dose increases will not have a greater analgesic effect. If the maximum dose has been given and the patient's pain control is inadequate, then the patient must be changed to another drug, the non-opioid supplemented with opioids, or adjuvant drugs added. This will probably involve moving up the analgesic ladder. Opioids, by contrast, have no ceiling to their analgesic effect – as long as side effects do not present a problem, then the dose of opioid can be increased until the pain is controlled. Dose titration is considered in more detail later.

Acetaminophen or paracetamol

Acetaminophen has analgesic and antipyretic (fever reducing) activity. It has no anti-inflammatory activity but does inhibit cyclo-oxygenase (see below) in the CNS. In most countries acetaminophen is freely available, without a prescription, and is widely used for the treatment of commonplace pains such as headache, toothache, etc. It is also effective for more serious medical conditions and is widely used, for example, post-operatively, for mild head and neck cancer pain and for bone pain. Acetaminophen has a 'morphine sparing effect' and can therefore be used to reduce the total dose of opioid required. It should not be omitted when progressing up the analgesic ladder (Kenner, 1994).

Acetaminophen does not cause gastric irritation but is hepatotoxic in high doses; sensitive individuals can be susceptible at lower doses. It should be used with great caution in patients with liver disease, and high doses may have untoward effects in individuals who consume large quantities of alcohol. Since it is a common ingredient in many over-the-counter treatments for colds, flu and general minor pains, care must be taken that the maximum dose is not exceeded, especially when several different preparations are being taken simultaneously. Its hepatotoxicity can cause death from delayed liver failure after severe overdose, such as suicide attempts; and patients 'rescued' from such an event should be given the antidote to acetaminophen poisoning, acetylcysteine.

Nefopam

Nefopam is effective for mild to moderate pain. It has no anti-pyretic or anti-inflammatory activity. Its mode of action is unclear, but it is thought to act centrally to reduce perception of pain. It is used for the relief of pain caused by injury, surgery and cancer. It may also be used for severe toothache. Nefopam may be an attractive alternative to opioids in that it does not cause respiratory depression or cause dependence. It does, however, have anticholinergic and sympathomimetic activity that can cause nausea, nervousness and a dry mouth. Because of its stimulatory action on the heart, it is not given to patients suffering from a heart attack and can cause dangerously elevated blood pressure when given with monoamine oxidase inhibitors (MAOIs).

Acetaminophen and nefopam are summarised in Table 7.1.

Non-steroidal anti-inflammatory drugs (NSAIDs)

All clinically useful NSAIDs are anti-inflammatory, antipyretic and analgesic. Because of these similarities, NSAIDs are traditionally grouped together as a single therapeutic entity but classified, and usually listed, according to their chemical structure. Although a table of these classifications is included here for completeness (Table 7.2), it has been suggested that such chemical grouping is trivial and clinically irrelevant (McCormack, 1994).

Tissue injury is associated with local release of various mediators including the prostaglandins (see Chapter 2). Prostaglandins (PGs) are thought not to mediate pain directly but to cause hyperalgesia by sensitising nerve endings to the effects of other mediators (McCormack, 1994). They are also involved in inflammation and fever. NSAIDs prevent these actions by stopping the synthesis of prostaglandins. This may explain why NSAIDs are less effective as analgesics in non-inflamed tissue.

NSAIDs are thought to act by inhibiting cyclo-oxygenase, a key enzyme in the pathway of synthesis of prostacyclin, prostaglandins and thromboxane from arachidonic acid (Figure 7.2). Arachidonic acid is a com-

Table 7.1 Acetaminophen and nefopam.

Drug	Uses	Dose	Side effects	Formulations
Acetaminophen	Headache, toothache, menstrual pains, colds, flue, migraine	Adults: 500 mg–1 g per dose. Doses 4–6 hourly. 3 month–1 year: 60–120 mg per dose. 1–5 years: 120–250 mg per dose. 6–12 years: 250–500 mg per dose. Doses 4–6 hourly to a max. of 4/24 hours.	Rarely nausea, rash, hepatotoxic in large doses, risk of overdose	Tablets, capsules, liquid, supositories
Nefopam	Injury, surgery, severe toothache, cancer pain	30–90 mg daily, 3 × daily when necessary.	Nausea, nervousness, dry mouth	Tablets, injection

Compiled from the *BMA Guide to Medicines and Drugs* and *MIMS.*
The manufacturer's SPC (summary of product characteristics) sheet should always be consulted for full prescribing information.

Table 7.2 Classification of NSAIDs.

Chemical class	Therapeutic agents
Salicylates	Aspirin
	Benorylate
	Difusinal
Acetates	Diclofenac
	Etodolac
	Indomethacin
	Sulindac
	Tolmetin
Propionates	Fenbrufen
	Fenoprofen
	Flurbiprofen
	Ibuprofen
	Ketoprofen
	Naproxen
	Tiaprofenic acid
	Ketorolac
Fenamates	Flufenamic acid
	Meclofenamate sodium
	Mefanamic acid
Oxicams	Piroxicam
	Tenoxicam
Pyrazolones	Azapropozone
	Phenylbutazone
Butazones	Nabumetone

Source: Doyle, D., Hanks, G.W.C. and MacDonald, N. (eds)
(1993) *Oxford Textbook of Palliative Medicine*. Reproduced by
permission of Oxford University Press.

ponent of cell membranes and thus ubiquitous – just which PGs are
produced varies in different tissues.

Individual NSAIDs have different modes of inhibitory activity on cyclo-
oxygenase; however, there is a relationship between the ability of an
NSAID to inhibit formation of these substances and their analgesic
properties.

PGs also have a protective role in the gastro-intestinal mucosa. The
action of NSAIDs on these PGs is not so welcome since they contribute
to the dyspepsia, peptic erosions or ulceration seen with these drugs.
Patients with previous ulcer disease are the most susceptible (Roth,
1988). Because of the untoward gastro-intestinal side effects, they are

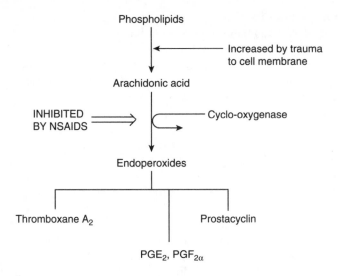

Figure 7.2   The cyclo-oxygenase pathway. Modified from Clarke R.S.J. (1990). Non-steroidal anti-inflammatory analgesics. *Current Opinion in Anasthesiology*, **3**, 607–611, Figure 1, with kind permission of International Thompson Publishing Services.

often given with food or in problematic cases with an antacid or histamine H_2 blockers.

The inhibition of synthesis of intrarenal vasodilatory prostaglandins is thought to be causative in the nephrotoxicity of these drugs (Cooper & Bennet, 1987). Patients at increased risk are the elderly, those with congestive heart failure, existing renal insufficiency, cirrhosis, low intravascular volume, or multiple myeloma. Patients receiving diuretics may also be at risk (Cooper & Bennet, 1987).

Perhaps the best known and most widely used NSAID is aspirin. A longstanding and commonly used analgesic, aspirin is used in a similar way to acetaminophen for 'everyday' pain. Aspirin is equianalgesic and has similar antipyretic activity to acetaminophen (Foster & Cox, 1983), the important difference between the two being that acetaminophen is not anti-inflammatory. These two analgesics are used more or less interchangeably by the general public; however, the use of aspirin during a viral infection has been implicated in the cause of Reye's syndrome in children. This condition, characterised by brain and liver damage is very rare, but still the association of aspirin with the disease has lead to aspirin being contraindicated in children under 12 years of age, except under close supervision as, for example, in Still's disease (juvenile rheumatoid arthritis). Acetaminophen should be used in preference to aspirin in children.

Another effect of aspirin is to reduce blood clotting, and it is given after heart attacks and as therapy to prevent blood clots.

NSAIDs come in a variety of formulations depending on the drug. Most are available as oral preparations and some may be given parenterally, rectally or topically. When given by mouth they are well absorbed, but all NSAIDs can cause gastro-intestinal irritation.

Adverse reaction reports in the UK would suggest that differences exist in the risk of gastro-intestinal reactions among the NSAIDs. Ibuprofen is considered to be associated with a lower risk than diclofenac, naproxen, indomethacin, ketoprofen and piroxicam. There is considerable inter-patient variation with different NSAIDs, and several may have to be tried before the one most suited to a particular patient is found.

More recently proprietary drugs have been developed which contain a mixture of an NSAID and a prostaglandin analogue which prevents the untoward gastro-intestinal side effects. Examples are the combination of diclofenac and misoprostil (Arthrotec) and naproxen with misoprostil (Napratec).

Topical applications of NSAIDs are most commonly used for joint pains. Used this way, they produce fewer side effects.

An overdose of salycilates results in salicylate toxicity, characterised by hyperventilation, tinnitus, sweating, abnormal breathing, biochemical disturbances and, in severe cases, convulsions and coma. Cognitive dysfunction may be associated with ibuprofen, indomethacin, naproxen and some other NSAIDs (Goodwin & Regan, 1982).

NSAIDs are widely used for back pain, menstrual pain, headaches, toothache, postoperative pain and soft tissue injuries. They are used in cancer patients and are the mainstay of pain relief in rheumatoid arthritis, osteoarthritis and gout, although they are without effect on the underlying disease process. As with side effects, responses to different NSAIDs vary between individuals, and it may be necessary to try a number of different agents before the one most suitable for a particular individual is found.

The commonly used NSAIDs are summarised in Table 7.3.

7.4　Opioid analgesics

The analgesic and euphoric properties of opiates were first discovered by the Chinese some 2000 years ago. Of all the opiates, morphine is the best known and most effective. Despite current sophisticated technology pharmacologists have not been able to improve upon nature, and opiates, isolated from the sap or latex of the opium poppy *Papaver somniferum*, remain the most powerful analgesics known to man – the opium poppy still being our greatest source of opiates. We now have a larger range of compounds available, since many synthetic derivatives of morphine, the opioids, have been produced, but they are all based on the natural compounds.

The term *opiate* is a specific term which describes drugs derived from the juice of the opium poppy. *Opioid* is a general term which includes naturally occurring, semisynthetic and synthetic drugs with opiate-like or morphine-like activity.

Morphine was isolated from the dried sap or latex of the opium poppy by Friedrich Sertürner (1783–1841), a young German chemist, in 1808. He noted its analgesic properties and the fact that it can induce a feeling of well-being and contentment. It can also induce hallucinations, and as well as dulling pain induce a state of narcosis – stupor or insensibility. This latter property gave the compound its name after Morpheus, the Greek god of sleep.

Throughout the nineteenth century morphine was widely used as a medication. By 1880 medical textbooks listed as many as 54 diseases that could be treated by morphine injection (Gray, 1991). Even then morphine was used for 'recreational' purposes, for the feelings it produced, and much morphine was consumed as 'laudanum'.

However, with its continued use, the habit-forming nature of morphine and the resultant physical dependence soon became apparent. By the end of the nineteenth century there were an estimated 250 000 addicts in the United States. Concern for this effect of morphine resulted in an act being passed in the US in 1906 which made it mandatory for medicines containing opium or alcohol to be clearly labelled with the contents and the words 'habit forming'. This was followed, in 1912, by the International Opium Convention, which restricted the trade in narcotic substances to medical and scientific use. Many agreements and treaties on narcotic use followed, the most important of which was the Single Convention on Narcotic Drugs in 1961 (amended, 1972). The pronouncements of this convention were adopted by 73 countries and are still in force today.

The Single Convention is the treaty that regulates the production, manufacture, import, export and distribution of narcotic drugs for medical use, with the aim of preventing the diversion of opioids from medicinal to illicit purposes. Countries which are a party to the Single Convention are required to control all aspects of opioid use within their territories and all international movement of opioids. In accordance with this convention reports on production, manufacture, movement and consumption of narcotics are made annually to the International Narcotics Control Board (INCB), situated in Vienna, Austria.

The fact that opioids are so firmly controlled adds to the public mis-

Table 7.3 Commonly used NSAIDs: Indications and doses.

Drug	Uses	Doses (adult dose)	Frequency	Side effects	Formulations
Aspirin	Colds, menstrual pains, headaches, joints, muscular aches	300–900 mg	4–6 hours	Nausea/vomiting, gastric bleeding, caution in children	Tablets, suppositories
Benorylate	Colds, flu, joint pain, menstrual pain, injury. Used with monitoring in juvenile arthritis	4–8 g daily	2–3 × daily after food	Nausea, constipation, indigestion	Tablets, liquid
Fenbrufen	Rheumatoid arthritis, osteoarthritis, gout, soft tissue injuries, surgery	900 mg daily	1–2 × daily after food	Nausea/vomiting, rash	Tablets
Ibuprofen	Rheumatoid arthritis, osteoarthritis, gout, moderate headache, menstrual pains, soft tissue injuries, after surgery	600–1.2 g daily (general) 1.2–2.4 g daily (arthritis)	4–6 × daily 3–4 × daily	Nausea/vomiting, heartburn/indigestion	Tablets, liquid, cream
Indomethacin	Rheumatoid arthritis, osteoarthritis, acute attacks of gout, ankylosing spondylitis, bursitis, tendinitis, patent ductus arteriosis	50–200 mg daily	1–2 × daily with food (slow release) 2–4 × daily (standard capsules)	Gastro-intestinal disorders, severe headache, dizziness	Tablets, liquid, injection, suppositories

WITHDRAWN

Drug	Uses	Dose	Frequency	Side effects	Preparations
Ketoprofen	Rheumatoid arthritis, osteoarthritis, ankylosing spondylitis, soft tissue injuries, gout, dysmenorrhoea	50–200 mg daily	2–4 × daily with food	Gastro-intestinal disorders, rash, hepatic or renal toxicity, bronchospasm	Tablets, sustained release capsules
Mefanamic acid	Headache, toothache, menstrual pains, excessive menstrual bleeding, rheumatoid arthritis, osteoarthritis	750 mg–1.5 g daily	3 × daily with food	Gastro-intestinal disorders, indigestion, nausea and vomiting	Tablets, capsules, liquid
Naproxen	Rheumatoid arthritis, osteoarthritis, ankylosing spondylitis, soft tissue injuries, gout, dysmenorrhoea	500 mg then 250 mg (menstrual cramp) 500–1250 mg (muscular pain and arthritis) 750 mg then 250 mg (gout)	6–8 hourly 1–2 × daily 8 hourly, all doses with food	Gastro-intestinal disorders, rash	Tablets, liquid, powder, suppositories
Piroxicam	Rheumatoid arthritis, osteoarthritis, ankylosing spondylitis, gout, bursitis, tendinitis, after surgery	10–40 mg daily	Once daily, with food	Nausea, indigestion, abdominal pain	Tablets, capsules, suppositories, gel

Compiled from the *BMA Guide to Medicines and Drugs* and *MIMS*.
The manufacturer's SPC (summary of product characteristics) sheet should always be consulted for full prescribing information.

conception that these are drugs to be avoided or even banned, but this is to misunderstand the purpose of the INCB. Although this body exists to regulate opioid use, it does not intend to restrict proper medical prescribing. The preamble of the convention states, 'The medical use of narcotic drugs continues to be indispensable for the relief of pain and suffering and ... adequate provision must be made to ensure availability of narcotic drugs for such purposes' (quoted in the WHO report, 1990).

Narcotic is another term used to describe morphine-like drugs and is derived from the Greek *narke* meaning torpor or numbness. The word narcotic can be confusing since it is used colloquially, and sometimes in legal terminology, to mean any drug which may be abused, such as cocaine or marijuana, which are not pharmacologically related to opioids. Herein lies the root of some of the problems of opioid use – confusion about the therapeutic role of opioids with their more unsavoury reputation as illicit street drugs. The fear of opioids or 'opiophobia' and the availability of opioids were discussed in greater detail in Chapter 5.

Opioid receptors

The existence of opioid receptors was first proposed in the early 1950s, but they were not characterised until the 1970s. The concept of receptors was mentioned in Chapter 2. In order to understand more fully the actions of opioids it is useful to know some more about receptor terminology.

Opioids are agonists at highly specific opioid receptors. These are divided into three types according to their different properties:

- μ (mu),
- κ (kappa),
- δ (delta).

These groups of opioid receptors have been further subdivided into μ_1, μ_2, κ_{1a}, κ_{1b}, κ_2, κ_3, δ_1 and δ_2. A fourth type of receptor was identified, called σ (sigma); but this is not a true opioid receptor, as actions mediated through this receptor are not antagonised by naloxone (Martin *et al.*, 1976).

Receptors are often defined in terms of the substances that act on that receptor. Thus the sigma receptor is not a true receptor since the biological actions produced by stimulation of this receptor subtype are not antagonised by naloxone. Antagonism by naloxone is one of the criteria used to establish a receptor as an opioid receptor.

The main responses mediated by the different opioid receptor types are listed in Table 7.4.

The majority of opioids are μ receptor agonists, with the result that they produce the side effects listed as well as analgesia. In theory, a pure δ agonist would be the ideal analgesic – pain control without side effects. The search for a δ agonist has yet to produce a therapeutically useful agent.

Table 7.4　Responses mediated by activation of opioid receptors.

Receptor	Response on activation	Natural ligand
μ (mu)	analgesia, respiratory depression, miosis, euphoria, reduced gastro-intestinal motility	β endorphin
κ (kappa)	analgesia, dysphoria, psychomimetric effects, respiratory depression	dynorphins
δ (delta)	analgesia	enkephalins

Agonists and antagonists

Messages are relayed between cells by one cell releasing a chemical 'messenger' which acts on another cell. The site of action is a specialised part of the cell – usually but not always the on the cell membrane – called a receptor. Anything which binds in a specific way to a receptor is termed a ligand. Something which 'sticks' non-specifically is not a ligand (your boots do not have mud receptors, but mud still sticks to them!).

Activation of a receptor produces a biological response – that is, the cell is prompted into action. If the ligand produces the normal biological response associated with that receptor, it is termed an agonist. If the ligand occupies the receptor without inducing any biological response, it is termed an antagonist (Figure 7.3). Going back to the lock-and-key analogy considered earlier (i.e. a receptor and ligand are like a lock and key – see Chapter 2) an agonist is like a duplicate key – it fits the lock and has the same effect as the real key. An antagonist is the wrong key – it goes into the lock but it won't turn, it won't open the lock and, more importantly, it will put that lock temporarily out of action. This can be a useful property to exploit. If the biological activity produced by receptor activation is something we don't want, the ability to block it or turn it off is very useful. So an antagonist will occupy the receptor, have no intrinsic activity of its own, and will prevent the activity of the natural agonist (Figures 7.3a and 7.3b).

Receptor binding is a dynamic event, and after the ligand has activated a receptor, the receptor-ligand complex will usually dissociate (the key comes out of the lock and leaves it free for another key to enter).

There are different types of antagonists. Antagonists may act in the same way as the natural ligand, and since the receptor–ligand complex is a dynamic structure, the natural ligand and the antagonist will be competing for the same receptor site (two keys competing for the same lock). Such a ligand is termed a competitive antagonist.

Some antagonists can bind so firmly to a receptor, usually by forming covalent bonds, that the reaction is not reversible (the wrong key is per-

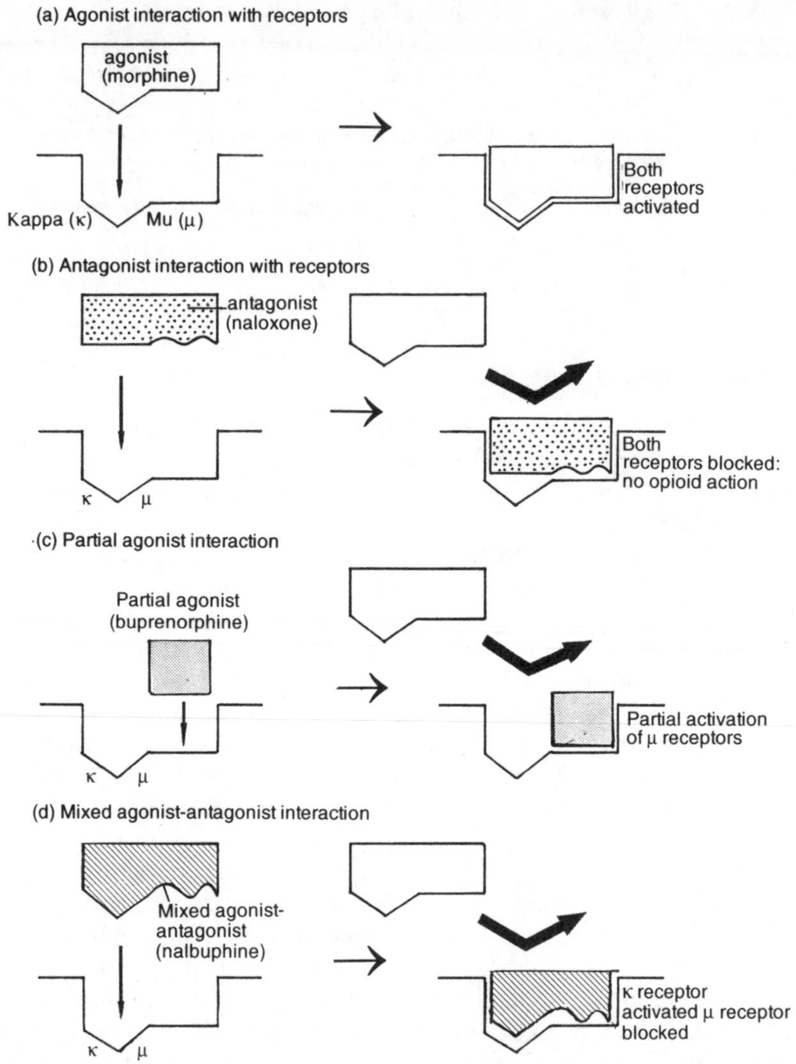

Figure 7.3 The different types of opioid receptors. (a) When an agonist interacts with both the mu and kappa receptors they are both activated. (b) When an antagonist (e.g. naloxone) blocks both receptors no opioid activity occurs. (c) When a partial agonist (e.g. buprenorphine) interacts with the mu receptor it activates the receptor, but does not have full activity. (d) When a mixed agonist-antagonist interacts with the receptor (e.g. nalbuphine) it activates the kappa receptor but blocks the mu receptor.

manently stuck in the lock). The receptor is then inactivated by what is termed a non-competitive antagonist.

Sometimes the activity at a receptor is not a clear cut 'all-or-none' event. For example, a compound may bind to the receptor, have a biological action, but have very low intrinsic activity at that receptor (it only partially opens the lock). The positive action of the compound on that receptor makes it an agonist, but no matter how much of the agent is used, the maximum biological response cannot be achieved. This type of agent is called a partial agonist. The commonest example of a partial opioid agonist is buprenorphine.

Because subsets of receptors exist, it is possible that a compound can act as an agonist at one receptor subtype while being an antagonist on another subtype. This is termed a mixed agonist-antagonist. Pentazocine, butorphanol and nalbuphine are important agonist-antagonists. Nalbuphine is a κ agonist and μ antagonist.

If a patient has been taking a pure opioid (an agonist) and has become physically dependant on the opioid, he/she will experience withdrawal symptoms if the opioid is suddenly stopped. What must also be remembered is that this withdrawal will also occur if a pure agonist is replaced by, or given with a drug that is only a partial agonist – or a mixed agonist-antagonist.

Thus buprenorphine, pentazocine, butorphanol or nalbuphine should never be given to patients who have been taking morphine or another strong opioid without taking this into consideration. These terms are summarised in Table 7.5.

Table 7.5 Definitions of ligands.

Type of ligand	Action
Agonist	Normal biological action – stimulates receptor
• Partial agonist	Normal biological action but has lower ceiling of effect. Will never achieve maximum biological response
Antagonist	Inhibits normal biological action – effectively blocks receptor
• Competitive antagonist	Competes for receptor site – thus block is not total or permanent
• Non-competitive antagonist	Remain covalently bound 'Permanently' blocks receptor
Mixed agonist-antagonist	Agonist at one receptor type while being antagonist at another type of receptor

Mechanism of action of the opioids

Opioids are predominantly agonists at μ receptors, which are quite widely distributed; $μ_1$ receptors are present in the brain and $μ_2$ receptors in the spinal cord. Morphine acts at all these different sites in the CNS, but the actions are complex.

Studies suggest that the brain is the predominant site of action after systemic administration of morphine (Pasternak, 1993). Receptor activation in the limbic system seems to lower or decrease the unpleasant response to pain – that is, morphine eliminates the subjective feeling of pain. Patients receiving morphine have reported that the pain remains but that it doesn't hurt anymore (Pasternak, 1993).

There are also morphine receptors in the periaqueductal grey, the raphe nucleus, locus coeruleus and nucleus reticularis gigantocellularis. All these areas are involved in the descending pathways of pain inhibition (see Chapter 2). Injection of morphine directly into any of these areas produces profound analgesia.

Morphine also has actions outside the brain. It has a direct action on pain transmission in the spinal cord by activation of μ receptors on spinal interneurons which causes hyperpolarisation of the interneurons and depression of pain transmission (Lipp, 1991). Morphine can also act indirectly by activating 'pain-modulating neurones' that project to the spinal cord, and this activation inhibits transmission from many primary afferent nociceptors to dorsal horn cells (Maruyama *et al.*, 1980). Thus the nociceptive pathway is not activated so markedly or not activated at all.

There is also some evidence that morphine can act peripherally to stop transmission of nociceptive signals even before they reach the spinal cord. Morphine injected intra-articularly following knee surgery elicits a profound analgesia without evidence of systemic absorption (Stein *et al.*, 1991).

Thus morphine is acting at several sites, peripheral, spinal and supraspinal, stopping transmission of nociceptive inputs, modulating nociceptive inputs or altering perception of nociceptive signals.

Morphine also interacts with adrenergic and serotoninergic neurones (see Chapter 2) and can have an enhanced effect on the descending pathways that inhibit the transmission of nociceptive signals.

Because of its wide spectrum of actions, morphine produces analgesia for a large range of painful conditions.

Clinically useful opioids

The opioids are commonly divided into weak and strong opioids. The commonly encountered opioids are listed in Table 7.6.

The selection of appropriate analgesic by using the WHO analgesic

Table 7.6   Commonly used opioid analgesics.

Weak opioids
  Codeine
  Dihydrocodeine
  Dextropropoxyphene
  Tramadol

Strong opioids
  Morphine
  Methadone ·
  Pethidine (meperidine)
  Hydromorphone
  Levorphanol
  Oxycodone
  Oxymorphone
  Diamorphine
  Fentanyl
  Sufentanil
  Papaveretum
  Dextromoramide
  Partial agonist
    Buprenorphine
  Agonist-antagonists
    Nalbuphine
    Butorphanol
    Pentazocine

ladder has been described. Below is a summary of the major features of each opioid.

Weak opioids

Codeine (methylmorphine) is the standard weak opioid analgesic. It binds to opioid μ receptors, but has low affinity. Codeine phosphate is well absorbed from the gastro-intestinal tract and is metabolised to nor codeine and morphine; this contributes significantly to its analgesic properties (Findlay *et al.*, 1978), although it is much less potent than morphine.

Codeine has analgesic, anti-tussive (suppresses coughing) and anti-diarrhoeal actions. It is an ingredient of many non-prescription cough syrups and cold relief preparations and is available 'over-the-counter' combined with aspirin as pain relief medication. It does not possess euphoric or addictive properties and hence is used widely by the public for headache, dysmenhorrea, muscular pain, etc. Constipation is a very common problem when taking codeine.

Dihydrocodeine is a semisynthetic analogue of codeine which also possess analgesic, anti-tussive and anti-diarrhoreal properties. Its analgesic potency is similar to, or sometimes slightly greater than, codeine.

Dihydrocodeine does appear to have a narrower therapeutic range than codeine, and there is a higher incidence of adverse effects as doses are increased. For example, increasing the dose from 30 to 60 mg will have marginal effect on analgesic activity but will greatly increase side effects (Inturrisi & Hanks, 1993). Thus dihydrocodeine does not have major advantages over codeine and may even have less flexibility in use.

Dextropropoxyphene is a synthetic derivative of methadone. It is a μ receptor antagonist with low receptor affinity. It is rarely given for anti-tussive or anti-diarrhoreal indications, although it does posses these actions.

Tramadol is a centrally acting opioid given by mouth or injection. It is claimed to produce less constipation and respiratory depression than conventional opioids. In cancer patients it has been shown to be less effective than modified-release oral morphine (Osipova *et al.*, 1991), although it is equally effective as pethidine for other painful conditions (labour pain, postoperative pain). It is a μ receptor agonist and also inhibits neuronal noradrenaline uptake and 5-HT release. Tramadol may be more easily available than other opioids in some circumstances, as it is not a controlled drug, although it still has abuse potential.

Strong opioids

Morphine is the main naturally occurring alkaloid of opium. It is the most widely known and used opiate and remains the 'gold standard' by which all other opioids are judged. It is available as the sulphate, tartrate or hydrochloride. Morphine acts spinally and supraspinally as an analgesic and alleviates and reduces the emotional reaction to pain. Patients frequently report that the pain is still present, but that they feel more comfortable.

Continuous dull pain is relieved more effectively than sharp, inter-mittent pain; but with sufficient morphine it is possible to relieve even the severe pain associated with renal or biliary colic (Reisine & Pasternak, 1996). Nociceptive pain is usually responsive to opioids although neu-ropathic pain may respond poorly and require higher doses of opioids (McQuay, 1988).

It generally produces euphoria, especially when injected, followed by a degree of sedation, lethargy and drowsiness, even sleep.

Morphine is available in three oral formulations; an elixir, an immediate release tablet and modified release tablets, of which there are several using different mechanisms of release.

Modified release preparations allow the drug to be delivered into the circulation slowly, over a period of 12–24 hours, rather than as a single bolus which occurs with immediate release tablets. Different preparations are called sustained release, continuous release or slow release.

Morphine is also available in parenteral (intravenous, intramuscular and intrathecal) and suppository forms. Doses of morphine must be titrated for each individual patient. This is covered in more detail below.

By acting on receptors in the gut morphine reduces gut motility and causes constipation. It releases histamine and may precipitate an asthma attack in susceptible individuals. Urticaria, itching and wheals may occur. Morphine can cause bile-duct or ureteral spasm exacerbating colic due to gall-stones or kidney-stones.

Morphine is metabolised to morphine-6-glucuronide (M-6-G) which although appearing in only small quantities binds to opioid receptors and produces potent opioid effects (Osborne *et al.*; Hanna *et al.*, 1990). M-6-G can accumulate in patients with renal insufficiency (Portenoy *et al.*, 1991; Sawe *et al.*, 1981; 1985) and can give rise to opioid toxicity. For this reason morphine should be used cautiously in patients with renal insufficiency.

Methadone is a synthetic opioid with a long half-life, of around 24 hours, which outlasts the duration of analgesic activity – around 4–6 hours. The result could be drug accumulation, this and a wide inter-patient variability in clearance make methadone difficult to monitor and complicates its long-term use in patients. Sedation, confusion and even death can occur if patients are not carefully monitored. Methadone clearance is also affected by other drugs that the patient may be taking, by disease state and renal function (Plummer *et al.*, 1988).

Methadone is most commonly encountered as maintenance therapy for drug addicts, since it prevents morphine euphoria and has lower addictive potential. However, is also used for non-malignant pain and in cancer patients, most usually those who are not responding to morphine.

Pethidine (meperidine) is less potent than morphine and has a shorter duration of action. It is widely used in surgery, as it is less likely than other opioids to cause spasms of smooth muscle. It is also used for analgesia in childbirth, although it can cause respiratory depression in the neonate. It causes restlessness rather than sedation and causes hyperthermia in patients who are receiving monoamine oxidase inhibitors (MAOIs), such as iponiazid, or tranylcypromine.

Repetitive dosing of pethidine can lead to accumulation of its toxic metabolite, norpethidine, giving rise to CNS hyperexcitability, which is characterised initially by subtle mood changes followed by anxiety, tremors, multifocal myoclonus and occasionally seizures.

Hydromorphone is a useful alternative in morphine intolerant patients. It has a short half-life, but is more potent than morphine. It is very soluble and is available in a concentrated dose form (10mg/ml) which can be injected in a very small volume. This may be useful under some circumstances, for example, with a cachexic patient. It is often the first-line strong opioid used in the elderly. Hydromophone is now available in a sustained release formulation, which can be used once every 12 hours. The hydromorphone is formulated as small white pellets contained within a gelatine capsule. Where patients are unable to swallow well, the capsule may be opened and the pellets sprinkled on to soft food. Hydromorphone is not available in the UK.

Levorphanol is a potent morphine derivative with a longer duration of action than morphine, but it must be used cautiously to avoid accumulation. It has a good oral:parenteral ratio of 1:2 (see below), although it is more sedating than morphine. It is less likely to produce nausea and vomiting and constipation and is therefore, for some patients, more acceptable than morphine.

Oxycodone is a synthetic derivative of morphine with an intravenous potency 1.5 times that of morphine, and an oral:parenteral ratio of 1:2 (see below). It is available in oral, rectal and injectable formulations. Compared with morphine it has a shorter duration of action, with the exception of suppositories which have analgesic activity over a slightly longer period than morphine (6–8h) and are the most commonly used form of this drug. Its availability as a combination preparation with non-opioids has led some people to believe, erroneously, that it is a weak opioid.

Oxymorphone is the metabolite of oxycodone, although it is available (in some countries) as an analgesic in its own right. There is no oral preparation of oxycodone, and it is usually given as a suppository or parenterally. Oxycodone has a similar pharmacokinetic profile to morphine. It does not have anti-tussive activity.

Diamorphine, diacetylmorphine or **heroin** is only available for legal medicinal use in the United Kingdom, Belgium and Canada. It is biotransformed to 6-acetylmorphine [6-MAM], which is hydrolysed to morphine and is therefore classified as a prodrug. Diamorphine is twice as potent as morphine (Kaiko *et al.*, 1981), and since both heroin and 6-MAM are more lipid soluble than morphine, they enter the brain more rapidly (Reisine & Pasternak, 1996). It is favoured by addicts as it gives a greater 'rush' (euphoria) and is considered by some to have a greater potential for addiction and dependence than morphine.

It is highly soluble, an advantage over morphine when parenteral administration in a small volume is required. However, this is also true for hydromorphone, which would be used in most countries (hydromorphone is not available in the UK). When given intravenously, diamorphine produces less gastro-intestinal effects, especially vomiting.

Fentanyl is closely related to pethidine and is 80–100 times more potent than morphine. Fentanyl is a general anaesthetic agent and is given combined with droperidol to produce 'neurolepalgesia' where analgesia and immobility occur without full loss of consciousness. This action can be reversed by naloxone leaving a tranquillised patient under the influence of droperidol alone. Fentanyl only became widely used as an analgesic with the introduction of transdermal patches (see route of administration of opioids, below). It is less likely to cause nausea and vomiting than morphine.

Papaveretum is a mixture of opium alkaloids, including papaverine, about 50% of which is morphine hydrochloride. Papaveretum has been in use for many years; however, in the last few years it has been reformulated to exclude one of the component, noscopine, which was found to be genotoxic (that is it can cause genetic mutation).

Dextromoramide is a potent μ agonist with a rapid onset of action and is twice as potent as morphine by mouth. It is short acting, and tolerance develops rapidly. With continued use its duration of action is attenuated from around 2 to 4 hours to only 1 or 2 hours (Inturrisi and Hanks, 1993). For these reasons it is unsuitable for long-term management of chronic pain but may be used for breakthrough pain.

Buprenorphine is a potent synthetic analgesic used postoperatively. It can be given by a variety of routes and is useful in patients who are unable to swallow since it can be given intranasally. It is a partial agonist and therefore has the potential to reduce analgesia or precipitate withdrawal effects in patients already taking opioids. It has a high affinity for opioid receptors and only dissociates slowly giving a long duration of action (6–8 hours) and lack of abstinence effects when stopped. There is an increased risk of psychomimetic side effects, and should respiratory depression occur, large doses of naloxone are required to reverse its action (Coyle *et al.*, 1995). It is not a treatment of choice in cancer patients.

Nalbuphine, butorphanol and **pentazocine** are all mixed agonist-antagonists. As such they all have the potential to precipitate withdrawal symptoms in patients already taking opioids who have developed physical tolerance. They are associated with a higher incidence of psychomimetic effects (agitation, confusion, dysphoria) than morphine (Coyle *et al.*, 1995).

Nalbuphine is a κ partial agonist, a weak μ antagonist and is slightly less potent than morphine. It has a similar duration of action and side effects profile to morphine. A potent analgesic when given by injection, it is not available as an oral formulation, which restricts its use. It has lower potential for abuse and in most countries is not a controlled drug.

Butorphanol is not available world-wide and only comes as a parenteral formulation.

Pentazocine is one-sixth to one-third as potent as morphine and closer in analgesic efficacy to aspirin and acetaminophen than the weak opioid analgesics. Respiratory depression is less than with other opioids, but there is a high risk of gastro-intestinal effects and rapid development of tolerance.

The strong opioid drugs are summarised in Table 7.7.

Parenteral:oral ratio

Opioids should be given by the least invasive route possible. Thus the oral route is preferred for most patients. However patients will, for a variety of reasons, be given infusions, intramuscular injections or spinal opioids. Rapid pain control may necessitate the use of injections which will be stopped in favour of oral treatment once the situation is controlled.

Changing from one route of administration to another involves an understanding of how doses of opioids given by these different routes are related. The parenteral:oral ratio defines the relative potency of an opioid given by a parenteral route to the oral route. The term parenteral in this context assumes that all parenteral routes are exactly the same, which is not strictly true – there are clearly differences between giving a drug by intramuscular or intravenous routes – however, for practical purposes the ratio can be used to convert doses. The important principle for clinical practice is that there is a difference in relative analgesic potency when the route of administration is changed and that adjustment of dose is necessary in order to achieve an equivalent effect, and to avoid any underdosing or toxicity.

When a drug is injected intravenously the total amount of drug is immediately available. An oral drug has to be absorbed, and it is the extent of absorption by the gastro-intestinal tract and factors such a first pass metabolism (see routes of drug administration) that will determine how much of the drug reaches the systemic circulation. If a drug is absorbed completely and not destroyed on passage through the liver, then its oral and intravenous potencies would be exactly the same. The parenteral:oral ratio would be 1:1.

If incomplete absorption or first pass metabolism halve the amount of drug that reaches the circulation, then twice as much of the drug must be given by the oral route to have the same circulating concentration as compared with the intravenous route. So if the plasma concentration after the oral dose is 1 (when half the drug has been 'lost') then this same amount of drug given parenterally would give a concentration of 2, hence the parenteral: oral ratio is 2:1.

Single dose studies showed the relative parenteral:oral potency of morphine to be 6:1 (Houde *et al.*, 1965). However, empirical clinical practice using chronically administered oral morphine in cancer patients has generated a ratio of 2:1 for the subcutaneous route or 3:1 for the intravenous route (Twycross, 1988; Hanks *et al.*, 1987). (By convention these figures are usually abbreviated to just 6, 2 or 3.) The discrepancy in these studies may be explained on the basis of important differences in methodology; the lower estimate was made in patients requiring a steady-state of pain relief, whereas the single dose estimate was made in patients with moderate to severe pain. In practice, the 6:1 ratio should be used in patients with acute pain, and for chronic administration the ratio of 3:1 is generally used when converting from parenteral to oral routes (Inturrisi & Hanks, 1993; Hanks *et al.*, 1996). The usual practice when converting from oral morphine to subcutaneous morphine (or diamorphine) is to divide the oral dose by two or three. The rectal to oral ratio for morphine is 1:1. The intramuscular:oral ratio for several opioids are given in Table 7.8.

Example: A patient's immediate pain has been controlled by morphine intramuscularly 50 mg every 4 hours. He is to be changed to oral drug. The parenteral:oral ratio for morphine is 4. Therefore the new dose would be 50 mg × 4 = 200 mg q 4 hr. The first oral dose would be given about 1 hour after the last im dose to allow the tablet to be absorbed before the last im dose was cleared.

An important point is that opioids will act more quickly when given intravenously than orally and less drug will be needed; but opioids are not 'better' and will not produce superior pain control when given intravenously – provided the equivalent dose is used.

When patients are changed from one route to another, it is the lack of attention to the route-dependant differences in dose that accounts for the common report of under-medication in cancer patients (Inturrisi & Hanks, 1993).

Equianalgesic doses

To aid comparisons and to enable patients to be switched from one drug to another, doses of different opioids are expressed as the dose that would be required to give the same analgesia as morphine. The conversion factor for levorphanol is 5, thus 50 mg of levorphanol would be needed to give the same analgesia as 10 mg of morphine. Table 7.9 lists the conversion factors for the commonly used opioids.

Example: A patient is to be changed from pethidine 200 mg every 6 hours to morphine every 6 hours. First calculate the total daily dose 200 × 4 = 800 mg. The conversion factor is 0.125, so the total daily dose of morphine is 800 × 0.125 = 100 mg. Given 6 hourly, this would be 100/4 = 25 mg morphine.

Table 7.7 Summary of some properties of the strong opioids.

Drug	Indications	Duration of action (hours)	Dose and frequency		Formulation
			Oral	Parenteral	
Morphine	Moderate to severe pain especially associated with cancer, or post-operative pain	4–5 (im, sc) 4–7 (po)	30 mg q 3–4 h Sustained release every 12 hours	10 mg q 3–4 h 90–129 mg	Oral – elixir, solution, tablets, sustained release tablets and capsules. Injection – iv, im, sc. Suppositories
Methadone	Moderate to severe pain especially for morphine-intolerant and post-operative pain. Used in withdrawal from dependence	4–5 (im, sc)	20 mg q 6–8 h	10 mg q 6–8 h	Oral – tablets, solution, linctus for cough
Pethidine	Moderate to severe pain	2–4	50 mg q 3–4 h	25–100 mg q 4h (sc/im) 25–50 mg iv	Oral – tablets, solution. Injection – im, sc, iv
Hydromorphone	Moderate to severe pain	4–5 (im, sc) 4–6 (po)	7.5 mg q 3–4 h Sustained release every 12 hours	1.5 mg q 3–4 h 4–24 mg	Oral – sustained release capsules. Injection – im, sc. Suppository
Levorphanol	Mild to moderate pain	4–8	4 mg q 6–8 h	1 mg q 6–8 h	Oral. Injections – im, sc

Oxycodone	Moderate to severe pain	4–6	30 mg q 3–4 h	—	Liquid, tablet, suppositories
Diamorphine	Moderate to severe pain	2–3	5–10 mg q 4 h		Oral – tablets, elixir. Injection – im, sc
Fentanyl	Moderate to severe pain. General anaesthetic	1–2	Initially 25 μg/h patch, titrate in 25 μg/h increments		Transdermal patch
Papaveretum	Moderate to severe pain	3–4		7–15 mg	Injection – im, sc
Dextromoramide	Moderate to severe pain particularly 'breakthrough' or 'incident' pain	2–3	up to 5 mg	up to 10 mg rectally	Oral – tablets. Injection – im, sc
Partial agonist					
Buprenorphine	Moderate to severe acute pain	6–9 (sub-lingual)	200–400 μg sublingually		Oral – tablets (sublingual)
Agonist-antagonist					
Nalbuphine	Moderately severe pain post-operative pain	2–4	10 mg	3–5 mg	Injection – im, sc, iv
Pentazocine	Moderately severe pain, labour pain, post-operative pain	2–4 (im)	25–100 mg q 3–4 h		Oral – capsules, tablets. Injection – im, sc, iv
Butorphanol	Moderate to severe pain	3–4			Injection – im, iv

Compiled from the *BMA Guide to Medicines and Drugs, MIMS*, or the literature.
The manufacturer's SPC (summary of product characteristics) sheet should always be consulted for full prescribing information.

Table 7.8 Parenteral: oral ratio for commonly used opioids.

Drug	Intramuscular/oral potency
Codeine	1.5
Morphine	6 – on repeat dosing 3
Hydromorphone	5
Methadone	2
Levorphanol	2
Diamorphine	(6–10)
Pethidine	4
Pentazocine	3
Oxycodone	2

Table 7.9 Conversion factors for calculating equianalgesic doses.

Drug	Conversion factor
Buprenorphine	50–60
Codeine	0.08
Dextromoramide	2
Dextropropoxyphene	0.16
Diamorphine	1
Dihydrocodeine	0.1
Hydromorphone	6–7.5
Levorphanol	5
Methadone	3–4
Oxycodone	1
Papaveretum	0.67
Pethidine	0.125
Pentazocine	0.06

Adapted from: Twycross & Lack (1989); Regnard & Tempest (1992).

Starting doses and dose titration

A patient who has had no more than limited exposure to opioids or who is totally naive should be started on a dose equivalent to 5 to 10 mg of morphine IM every 4 hours. The dose should then be titrated to the level of pain. Some patients will need special considerations when choosing the starting dose. Specifically those patients:

- with renal impairment;
- who have been taking opioids previously (whether for therapeutic reasons or as opioid abusers);
- with a history of alcohol abuse.

Where there is renal impairment, either due to disease or because the patient is elderly, the starting dose should be reduced since the metabolite morphine-6-glucuronide is more likely to accumulate.

If patients have been taking the prescribed opioid previously, they may well have developed some tolerance and will need a higher starting dose. However, if they have been taking a different opioid from the one which is to be administered, this is not the case. The cross-tolerance between different opioids is not complete, and patients who are switched from one opioid to another should be started on the new opioid at one-third to one-half the equianalgesic dose of the original drug.

Similarly patients with a history of alcohol abuse display tolerance to opioids and may well need higher starting doses of opioids or more rapid dose escalation.

The aim of dose titration should be to provide effective pain control and minimal side effects, employing the lowest dose of opioid which will achieve this result. Dose adjustment may take several days and doses will need to be reviewed as part of the ongoing process of monitoring the patient. If the starting dose is inadequate, it should be increased by one-quarter to one-half. The majority of patients will be given a rapidly available oral formulation or intravenous drug every four hours. Since there is no ceiling to analgesic activity, titration may result in final doses of up to several hundred milligrams every four hours. The dose of morphine may range from 2.5 mg 4-hourly to 2500 mg 4-hourly, and there are anecdotal reports of much higher doses (Inturrisi & Hanks, 1993). This dose-range of a thousand-fold difference is remarkable and not seen with any other medication. An algorithm for the titration of post-operative pain is given in Gould *et al.* (1992).

Where tolerance develops, the efficacy of the opioid may start to decline and doses will need to be increased or the drug changed to a different opioid. Increasing doses may also signal disease progression.

Maintaining adequate analgesia

Initially morphine was given on a PRN (when needed) basis. This can be useful if the aim is to titrate the dose, but for continued pain relief it is generally inefficient; the patient suffers pain and makes a request before the next dose of drug is given. The pain is controlled but then the analgesic wears off and pain returns. What is happening is that plasma levels of drug are fluctuating widely in a pattern of 'peaks and troughs' (Figure 7.4a). In order to overcome these problems a regular dosing schedule was devised whereby routine administration of morphine every 4 hours kept plasma levels within a critical range that provided adequate pain control (Figure 7.4b).

Four-hourly drug administration is inconvenient, especially at night,

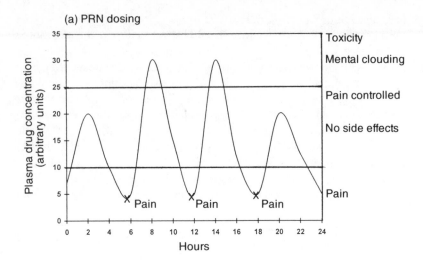

(a) PRN dosing

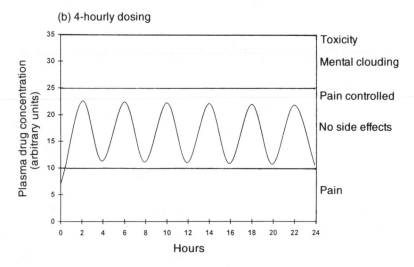

(b) 4-hourly dosing

Figure 7.4 Changes in plasma opioid levels in relation to therapeutic efficacy after different dosages of morphine. When given on a prn basis (a) pain occurs as the effect of the morphine wears off. A high dose will then be required to control the pain, taking plasma concentrations high enough to cause side effects. This pattern is then repeated. If, however, doses are given on a regular basis (b) then pain can be controlled and side effects avoided.

and particularly intrusive for patients in palliative care or those requiring long-term use of analgesics. These problems were addressed with the introduction of modified release preparations which, by incorporating the morphine into a sustained release tablet, or capsule, delivers a constant dose of drug over several hours. Immediate release morphine reaches its peak concentration at around 0.25–1.0 hours, whereas modified release formulations usually take 2–4 hours to reach their peak concentration. The duration of analgesia is around 4 hours for immediate release morphine and 12 hours for modified release preparations (Hanks *et al.*, 1996).

The total daily dose of morphine remains the same whatever type of formulation is used, so the total daily dose of morphine that the patient receives is calculated and this is divided by the number of modified release tablets.

Example: A patient is to be changed from 50 mg morphine every 4 h to a modified release capsule. Total daily morphine = 50 × 6 = 300 mg. For two modified release capsules to be given daily, the dose would be 300/2 = 150 mg per capsule.

Modified release morphine has been a very welcome development in the control of continuous pain and especially cancer pain. Patients are more likely to comply with the recommended dosing regimen, thus giving superior pain management. In one study it was found that patients took 54% of the prescribed dose of short-acting analgesics compared with 92% of the prescribed long-acting analgesics. The authors concluded that the long-acting analgesic provided longer periods of comfort, was more convenient to take and did not interrupt sleep (Rolling Ferrell, 1991). Modified release preparations of morphine have also been shown to improve patients' quality of life (Ferrell *et al.*, 1989). In some countries hydromorphone is also available as a modified release preparation.

Changing the route of administration may require some adaptation on the part of the patient. For example, an oral drug has a slower onset of action than parenteral formulations. In changing to oral therapy it may be better to gradually reduce parenteral doses and simultaneously increase oral doses over a few days.

All continuous dosing regimens, whether modified release or constant infusion, are likely to need supplementation with more rapidly acting preparations for breakthrough pain.

Example: A patient is receiving 200 mg of pethidine orally every 4 hours. He is to be changed to the new modified release morphine.

- First calculate his daily dose of pethidine: 200 mg × 6 = 1200 mg.
- Calculate the equianalgesic dose of morphine – the conversion factor for pethidine is 0.125. Thus, 1200 mg × 0.125 = 150 mg.
- The total daily dose would be given as two modified release capsules every 12 hours. Thus 75 mg morphine sustained release q 12 hours.

Opioid responsiveness of pain

Many pains respond in a predictable way to analgesic drugs, and recent studies have shown that using guidelines, notably the WHO analgesic ladder, up to 90% of cancer pain can be controlled with oral analgesic drugs (Hanks *et al.*, 1993). Evidence also shows that a substantial sub-population of patients with chronic non-malignant pain can obtain sustained analgesia, without toxicity, from opioids (Portenoy, 1990). The main reason for incomplete control is often cited as lack of knowledge of analgesic use and a consequent underdosing for the condition. There are, however, some types of pain that are either not responsive to opioids or, more properly, are not best managed with opioid analgesics.

The identification of pain that was not controlled by opioid drugs lead to the term 'opioid non-responsive pain' being used. Classically it was pain of neuropathic origin that was thought to be unresponsive to opioid drugs. This view has been challenged, however, by authors who consider that frequently the opioids have not been taken to a high enough level before classifying the pain as non-responsive (Portenoy *et al.*, 1990).

Opioid drugs have no 'ceiling' to their analgesic activity – that is, the higher the dose given, the greater the analgesia. What limits how much drug is given are the side effects associated with the particular opioid. Thus, when opioids are used they should be titrated to the individual patient and a dose identified which produces effective analgesia with acceptable side effects or side effects easily manageable with other medication.

It may be more useful, therefore, not to talk about 'opioid non-responsive pain' but to classify such pain as that which is not best managed by opioids, since the dose required produces unacceptable side effects. However, it must be remembered that the balance between effective analgesia and unwanted toxicities in the case of oral morphine is usually weighted very much towards analgesia (Hanks *et al.*, 1993).

7.5 Adjuvant analgesics

Strictly speaking, an adjuvant drug is one that potentiates the activity of another drug, but the term has also come to mean a drug that assists treatment of the condition. For example, an adjuvant anxiolytic may be given alongside an analgesic to reduce anxiety; this will undoubtedly help pain relief even though the anxiolytic is not having a direct pharmacological action on the analgesic. An adjuvant analgesic probably has a primary indication other than pain, but has proved useful in controlling pain. Although adjuvant analgesics usually have an indirect action in pain relief by ameliorating some other condition, they can sometimes control pain directly. They are sometimes called 'co-analgesics', and these drugs are usually, but not always, administered in combination with one or more of the primary analgesics, which may be an NSAID and/or an opioid.

The usefulness of an adjuvant drug will depend on the cause of the pain or the existence of some other symptom concurrent with the pain. Any differences the drug may display must be appreciated – for example, in dosing or duration of action when it is employed as an analgesic as compared to when it is used for its primary indication. It is also important that patients who may encounter these drugs under other circumstances appreciate their use in pain control. For example, a patient with a rather elusive pain, with no obvious cause, may be given imipramine. If he then discovers that imipramine is an antidepressant, he may feel 'let-down', disappointed that his pain is not being believed and he is being fobbed-off with antidepressants because the healthcare team obviously think his pain is not real. A simple explanation from the nurse of the dual role of this drug would do much to avoid this response.

Since the analgesic dosing has often not been investigated for many of these drugs, it may be advisable to start with a relatively low dose and titrate upwards. Attention must also be paid to side effects, as it is clearly undesirable to induce side effects which exacerbate some aspect of the patient's condition. Additive or unpredictable side effects can sometimes occur when a patient is receiving a 'cocktail' of medication.

The main drugs used for adjuvant analgesia are listed in Table 7.10. The indications and doses of the more commonly used drugs are summarised in Table 7.11.

Antidepressants

Antidepressant drugs have been shown to be analgesic for a wide variety of painful conditions including:

- headache,
- migraine,
- arthritis,
- low back pain,
- postherpetic neuralgia,
- fibromyalgia,
- diabetic neuropathy,
- chronic facial pain,
- psychogenic pain.

The analgesic dose is usually lower than that required for antidepressant actions, and the onset of analgesia is quicker. This suggests that these drugs have intrinsic analgesic activity and are not merely counteracting depression. It has also been shown that analgesia can occur even if mood is

Table 7.10 Adjuvant analgesic drugs.

Class	Examples
Antidepressants	
Tricyclic antidepressants	amitriptyline, clomipramine, desipramine, doxepin, imipramine, nortriptyline
Newer antidepressants	maprotiline, trazodone
Monoamine oxidase inhibitors	phenelzine, tranylcypromine
Anticonvulsants	carbamazepine, clonazepam, phenytoin, valproate
Oral local anaesthetics	flecainide, mexiletine, tocainamide, ketamine
Neuroleptics	fluphenazine, haloperidol, methotrimeprazine, pimozide
Muscle relaxants	carisoprodol, chlorzoxazone, cyclobenzaprine, methocarbamol orphenadrine, baclofen, diazepam
Smooth muscle relaxants	alverine, dicyclomine, mebeverine, hyoscine, propantheline
Antihistamines	hydroxyzine
Psychostimulants	caffeine, dextroamphetamine methylphenidate, pemoline
Corticosteroids	dexamethasone, methylprednisolone, prednisolone
Sympatholytic drugs	phenoxybenzamine, prazosin
Calcium-channel blockers	nifedipine
Miscellaneous	capsaicin, clonidine, L-tryptophan

Modified from Portenoy (1993).

not altered. Antidepressants may act by inhibiting noradrenaline re-uptake and by stimulating descending pathways in the spinal cord to increase release of endogenous analgesics.

These drugs are especially useful in cases of neuropathic pain and they can have a morphine-sparing effect (that is, when given together with morphine, a lower dose of morphine can be used to give comparable analgesia). They are useful for patients with depression and insomnia.

Tricyclic antidepressants and monoamine oxidase inhibitors (MAOIs) are dangerous in overdose; tricyclics can produce coma, cause fits and disturb heart rhythm, MAOIs can cause fits. Both types of drug should be used with caution in patients with cardiovascular disease.

Table 7.11 Adjuvant analgesics: indications and doses.

Indication	Preferred drugs	Dosing schedule	Starting dose (mg/day)	Usual daily dose (mg/day)	Comment
Antidepressants					
Continuous neuropathic pain. Pain complicated by depression or insomnia	amitriptyline, doxepin, imipramine, desipramine, nortryptyline, paroxetine	qrh	10–25	50–150	Amitriptyline preferred. If toxicity too great, try desipramine, nortryptyline or paroxetine.
Anticonvulsants					
Lancinating neuropathic pain	carbamazepine, phenytoin, valproate	q 6–8 h qhs q 8 h	200 300 500	600–1600 300 750–2250 or higher	Baclofen is not an anti-convulsant, but has potential efficacy in lancinating pain and thalmic pain.
	clonazepam, baclofen	q 12 h q 8 h	0.5 15	2–7 30–60 or higher	
Oral local anaesthetics					
Neuropathic pain	mexiletine, tocainide	q 8 h q 8 h	300 600	450–900 1200–1800	Mexiletine is safer than tocainide and should be tried first.

Contd.

Table 7.11 *Contd.*

Indication	Preferred drugs	Dosing schedule	Starting dose (mg/day)	Usual daily dose (mg/day)	Comment
Neuroleptics					
Pain complicated delerium or nausea; refractory neuropathic pain	fluphenazine, haloperidol, methotrimeprazine	q 8 h q 6–12 h q 6 h	2 2 20	3–6 2–10 20–60	Not first line. Potential by toxicity. Methotrimeprazine is proven analgesic, useful for terminal pain and agitation.
Muscle relaxants					
Acute musculoskeletal pain	carisoprodol, chlorzoxazone, methocarbamol, cyclobenzaprine	q 6 h q 6–8 h q 6 h q 8 h	800 750 4000 30	800–1200 750–1200 4000 30	Mechanism of action unknown.
Smooth muscle relaxants					
Gut spasms and IBS	alverine, dicyclomine, mebeverine, hyoscine, propantheline	tds before meals tds before meals tds before meals q 8 h q 8 h		60–120 30–60 375 80 45–100	
Antihistamines					
Pain complicated by anxiety or nausea	hydroxyzine	q 6–8 h	75	200	Hydroxyzine analgesic in controlled trials with high parenteral doses. No evidence of analgesia from oral doses.

Indication	Drug	Schedule	Starting dose	Dose range	Comments
Corticosteroids Pain from infiltration of neural structures; bone pain; pain in patients with far advanced cancer	dexamethasone	q 6–8 h	10–20 then 1–2 q 12 h or lower/higher depending on need	2–24	Higher doses used in cord compression.
Analeptics To reduce opioid-induced sedation	methylphedate, dextroamphetamine, pemoline	2/day 2/day 2/day	5 5 17.5	10–40 10–40 17.5–75	Higher doses sometimes.
Bisphosphates Bone pain	pamidronate, etidronate, sodium clodronate	divided doses once daily 2/day	15 5 mg/kg	15–60 10 mg/kg 1600	Inhibit osteoclast activity. Need to monitor blood calcium, phosphate, magnesium and potassium.
Radiopharmaceuticals Bone pain from metastases	strontium-89, rhenium-186	once daily		1–2 MBq/kg 1000 MBq	Absorbed at areas of high bone turnover. Marrow toxicity mild.

Modified from Coyle et al. (1995).
The manufacturers' SPC (summary of product characteristics) should be consulted for full information on any drug mentioned in this table.

Anticonvulsants

Anticonvulsant drugs are useful for the treatment of neuropathic pain. They are especially effective for controlling lancinating neuropathic pain (Swerdlow, 1984) and other types of episodic neuropathic pains. They have proved useful in trigeminal and glossopharyngeal neuralgias, postherpetic neuralgia, post-traumatic neuralgia, the so-called 'flashing' dysaesthesias in patients with spinal cord injury and painful diabetic neuropathy. Baclofen may be used intraspinally for refractory spasticity. It has also been used for lancinating pain and the treatment of trigeminal neuralgia.

The mechanism of action of the anticonvulsants is not known but may involve suppression of paroxysmal discharges in the nervous system and a reduction of neuronal hyperexcitability.

Oral local anaesthetics

Analgesia can be demonstrated in patients with post-operative pain and various chronic pain syndromes, including neuropathic pains after brief intravenous infusions of anaesthetics. The advent of oral local anaesthetics gave the opportunity of evaluating these drugs in pain syndromes. Tocainide has been shown to be effective in patients with trigeminal neuralgia, and flecainide has been demonstrated to be effective in cancer patients with painful malignant infiltration of nerves. These agents may be useful for both lancinating and continuous dyasthesias.

More recently ketamine has been proposed for the prevention and treatment for chronic persistent pain (Coe, 1997).

Neuroleptics

Few studies have shown positive effects of neuroleptics alone on pain, although chlorpromazine has been demonstrated to be effective in thalamic pain. Haloperidol has been used in painful neuropathy.

Neuroleptics have proved more useful in combination with antidepressants or opioids. An opioid-sparing effect has been noted in cancer patients (Breivik & Rennemo, 1982).

Some neuroleptics have proved useful in bedridden cancer patients where pain is associated with anxiety, nausea or restlessness. Chlorpromazine, haloperidol and prochlorperazine have anti-emetic activity and may help patients who have nausea and vomiting.

Corticosteroids

Coticosteroids are used in patients with bone pain, spinal cord compression, raised intra-cranial pressure, visceral pain and advanced cancers. They can reduce oedema and thereby relieve pressure on compressed structures. Corticosteroids have an anti-inflammatory activity. The analgesic activity is also accompanied by an increase in appetite, and a beneficial effect on mood and malaise in these patients. Just how corticosteroids achieve this effect is unknown, but they are often reported to induce a 'feeling of well-being'. Dexamethasone has anti-emetic and anti-nausea actions and may help patients with persistent nausea.

Corticosteroids are also used to treat certain conditions such as skin lesions or inflammatory bowel disease where their curative action also provides pain relief.

Antihistamines

Antihistamines can have analgesic effects, although they are best employed in patients who have other indications for antihistamines, such as itch or nausea. They are mildly sedating and this may be beneficial in some patients.

Benzodiazepines

Both diazepam and midazolam have been shown to bring pain relief and are especially useful in patients with high levels of anxiety or insomnia. Benzodiazepines can also reduce muscle spasms.

Muscle relaxants

Diazepam is the only muscle relaxant to have an appreciable effect in actually relaxing skeletal muscle. Muscle relaxants have been shown to be analgesic in action; however their mechanism of action is unknown. They are usually given for acute musculoskeletal pain. Drugs which act on smooth muscle, such as hyoscine, dicyclomene, pirenzipine, mebeverine, alverine and propantheline may be given to relieve painful spasms of the gut or for treatment of conditions such as irritable bowel syndrome (IBS). These drugs may, however, cause anticholinergic side effects, such as dry mouth or blurred vision.

Calcitonin

Calcitonin is used in patients with bone pain, especially in cases refractory to NSAIDs and corticosteroids. Calcitonin is a naturally occurring hormone, produced by the thyroid gland, that promotes deposition of calcium in bone. In cancer patients a synthetic form is given to reduce osteoporosis and reduce the elevated plasma levels of calcium that occur in patients with bone cancer or bony metastases. As well as relieving pain calcitonin may help to alleviate nausea and vomiting which can be caused by high plasma calcium. Its use has declined since the introduction of bisphosphonates.

Bisphosphonates

Bisphosphonates include etidronate sodium, sodium didronate, pamidronate disodium and tiludronic acid. They prevent bone reabsorption by inhibiting osteoclast activity and dissolution of sodium apatite crystals. They are used for tumour-induced hypercalcaemia and bone pain associated with metastases especially in cancer of the breast, multiple myeloma or Paget's disease. Bisphosphonates are also used for the treatment and prevention of osteoporosis, especially in postmenopausal women.

Capsaicin

Experimentally capsaicin can reduce the level of peptides such as substance P in small diameter primary afferent neurones. This has led to the investigation of topical capsaicin for treatment of pain, although its efficacy is debatable. It has been prescribed for the relief of post-herpetic neuralgia, rheumatoid arthritis, oesteoarthritis and painful diabetic neuropathy. In one study of patients with post-herpetic neuralgia up to one-third of patients benefited from topical capsaicin (Watson *et al.*, 1988).

Sympatholytic drugs and nifedipine

Sympathetically maintained pain is often treated by nerve blocks but may also respond to treatment with phenoxybenzamine or nifedipine.

7.6 Topical anaesthetics

Topical anaesthetics may be applied to the skin to relieve an existent pain or to anaesthetise an area of skin before a minor surgical procedure. Many over-the-counter preparations for wasp and bee stings or minor skin abrasions such as cuts and burns contain low concentrations of topical anaesthetics. Treatments for haemorrhoids contain local anaesthetics, such as lignocaine, often in combination with a topical steroid to relieve inflammation. To reduce absorption of the anaesthetic into the circulation a vasoconstricting agent may also be included, which also helps reduce the haemorrhoid and relive pain.

An EMLA (Eutectic Mixture of Local Anaesthetic) is a cream which is applied to the skin to produce anaesthesia before minor surgical procedures including venepuncture or intravenous cannulation. It contains lidocaine and prilocaine both at a concentration of 25 mg/g. Approximately 2 g of EMLA cream should be applied about 1 hour before commencement of the procedure. Its effect lasts about 5 hours (for review see Buckley & Benfield, 1993).

7.7 Drugs for specific pain conditions

Angina

There are three classes of drug used to treat anginal pain: nitrogylcerines, beta-blockers and calcium channel blockers. The nursing aspects of these drugs and education for patients using them are reviewed by Gleeson (1991).

Nitroglycerines

Nitroglycerine has been the treatment for anginal pain for more than a hundred years, and although several nitrate derivatives are now available, nitroglycerine remains the standard by which other nitrates are judged. Nitrates relieve both exertional and vasospastic angina, but their exact mechanism of action has not been elucidated. All nitrates work by dilating the venous capacitance vessels, which reduces venous return to the heart and thus reduces the preload on the heart. In larger doses nitroglycerine dilates arterioles, decreasing systemic vascular resistance, which slightly decreases afterload. A combination of reducing preload and afterload lessens the heart's work load and therefore decreases the myocardial oxygen demand.

Preload is the blood volume returning to the heart. If this is increased the heart has to work harder to cope. Afterload is the pressure from the aorta and peripheral vasculature that resists the ejection of blood from the ventricles during the systole.

Nitroglycerine also dilates coronary arteries, improving the oxygen supply to the myocardium (heart muscle) especially to ischaemic areas.

Nitrates are available as a number of compounds and in a wide variety of formulations: sublingual, buccal and oral tablets; sublingual sprays; sustained release tablets and capsules; chewable tablets; transmucosal ointment and patches, and intravenous solutions. The glycerine trinitrate in tablets is chemically unstable, and storage is therefore very important. Tablets should be kept in a dark glass container with a foil-lined cap and without any cotton wool wadding. The tablets should be discarded after 8 weeks regardless of how they have been stored. The choice of formulation will depend upon the patient's condition.

Emergencies may be treated by intravenous injection of a solution, as this is most rapidly acting. Acute attacks of angina, that are not life threatening, are generally aborted by use of oral glyceryl trinitrate, in the form of sprays, sublingual, buccal or chewable tablets. The relief of pain after using these preparations is almost immediate. Patients who are at risk of developing angina post-operatively may also be given intravenous nitroglycerine.

Long-term prophylactic management of angina employs long acting agents such as:

- glyceryl trinitrate,
- penyaerythritol tetranitrate,
- isosorbide dinitrate,
- isosorbide mononitrate.

These agents are usually given as sustained release capsules or for glyceryl trinitrate as transdermal patches or ointment, although the oral, buccal and sublingual routes can still be employed.

The vasodilatory action of nitrates gives rise to their most common side effect – facial flushing and headache. Both effects are greatest at the start of treatment and diminish with time. They can be avoided by dose titration to the individual patient. Tolerance and cross tolerance to nitrates can develop with continued use.

Beta-blockers

Beta-blockers are effective in reducing the frequency and severity of exertional angina. They are not useful for vasospastic angina and may even exacerbate the condition. Beta-blockers block the sympathetic drive to the heart, by acting on beta receptors on the myocardium. These receptors normally respond to catecholamine stimulation by increasing contractility and heart rate. By preventing these responses, beta-blockers reduce the work that the heart is allowed to perform, and the oxygen demand, to a level which is below that which would provoke an anginal attack. They are used prophylactically to prevent anginal attacks. Cardioselective beta-blockers are:

- acebutol,
- atenolol,
- bisopropolol,
- metopropolol.

The non-cardioselective blockers may produce bronchospasm. These include:

- nadolol,
- oxprenolol,
- pindolol,
- propranolol,
- sotalol,
- timolol.

Both cardioselective and non-cardioselective blockers have similar side effects of: fatigue and lethargy; reduced heart rate; reduced systolic blood pressure; depressed myocardial contractility; bronchospasm; hypoglycaemia; loss of libido, and sensitivity to cold.

Calcium channel blockers

Calcium channel blockers can be used to treat both exertional and vasospastic angina. Calcium causes the myocardial and vascular smooth muscle to contract. Depolarisation of cells causes a rapid influx of sodium followed by a slower influx of potassium. The strength of both cardiac and smooth muscle contraction is related to the calcium concentration. Calcium channel blockers inhibit calcium inflow into cells, resulting in a more controlled and efficient contraction of the cardiac muscles. This consumes less energy, requires less oxygen and reduces afterload. Coronary vasodilatation allows more oxygenated blood to perfuse the myocardium.

Calcium channel blockers have been classified by the WHO according to their pharmacological and clinical effects:

- Class I: verapamil;
- Class II: amlodipine; nicardipine; nifedipine;
- Class III: diltiazem.

Class I drugs have depressant action on cardiac contraction and may precipitate heart failure if there is AV or SA node dysfunction or if beta-blockers are given concurrently. Class II drugs do not have this effect and may be prescribed with beta-blockers provided the patient is closely monitored. Nifedipine can be given sublingually for an acute attack of angina pectoris.

Calcium channel blockers lower blood pressure and heart rate. The patient's cardiovascular status must, therefore, be carefully monitored. Hypotension and bradycardia are most likely when therapy begins, when dose is increased and when other antihypertensive or cardiac medications are added. Patients should be taught to monitor their own heart rate and told to contact the hospital or other healthcare unit when their heart rate falls below 60 beats per minute or if they feel their heart pounding. Hepatic and renal function may also be impaired by calcium channel blockers.

Migraine

As discussed in Chapter 3, migraine is essentially a severe unilateral headache often accompanied by nausea and/or vomiting. Conventional treatment, therefore, involves analgesics plus anti-emetics. Because it is a recurrent condition, migraine is also managed by giving prophylactic medication to circumvent recurrence.

Treatment

Usually aspirin, paracetamol or codeine are given for the pain of migraine. Many preparations designed specifically for migraine contain both paracetamol and codeine. Where these are ineffective an NSAID can be used. Since nausea and vomiting can prevent gastric absorption of the analgesics, a suppository form of these drugs can be used, although many patients do not like this route of administration. Metoclopramide or domperidone are the usual anti-emetics for nausea and vomiting.

Caffeine has been used for many years to prevent the development of headache when the early warning symptoms are present. Ergotamine, a more powerful analgesic drug, is also used with caffeine once the headache has started in patients who do not respond to simple analgesics. Ergotamine is most effective when given during the early phase of the attack (within 60–90 minutes of onset) and can actually exacerbate symptoms if given later. It produces generalised constriction of blood vessels throughout the body and therefore should not be prescribed for patients with poor circulation. If taken frequently it can seriously reduce the circulation in the hands and feet.

The vascular changes in migraine are thought to be mediated by serotonin which has lead to the search for a serotoninergic drug for migraine. Sumatriptan is a 5-HT_{1D} agonist which is though to act by constricting the dilated intracranial vessels. It can be given by injection, which is useful where active vomiting is present, or by tablet. A single dose can relieve migraine headache at any stage of the attack; the injection produces relief in 10–15 minutes, the tablet in 30 minutes. It should be avoided in patients with ischaemic heart disease, previous myocardial infarction, Prinzmetal's angina, coronary vasospasm or coronary artery disease. It must not be given within 72 hours of administration of ergotamine. Not every patient responds to sumatriptan.

Prophylaxis

Patients who have two or more attacks of migraine a month or who respond poorly to acute therapy are often given prophylactic medication. Two main groups of drugs are used: beta-blockers and serotonin antagonists.

The beta-blockers most commonly used are:

- metoprolol,
- nadolol,
- propranolol,
- timolol.

These drugs are thought to have effects on the cranial vasculature. They have been discussed above (see: Angina pectoris).

The 5-HT $_{1 \text{ and } 2}$ receptor antagonists used prophylactically are:

- pizotifen,
- methysergide,
- cyproheptadine.

These drugs inhibit vasodilatation. Treatment with the agents should not exceed 6 months without a 1-month drug-free interval. This is also a sensible measure to see how the patient is progressing since migraine can resolve spontaneously. The side effects of these drugs are summarised in Table 7.12.

Childbirth

It is common practice to avoid drugs wherever possible during pregnancy and this caution extends in to the period of actual childbirth. Analgesic drugs can cross the placenta and affect the fetus, so agents such as opioids are avoided. The most widely used methods of pain control for the women in labour are entonox (gas and air) or epidural anaesthesia. This latter technique is covered below under spinal administration of drugs.

Entonox is a gaseous mixture of 50% oxygen and 50% nitrous oxide which acts as an analgesic when inhaled. It is used for other procedures besides childbirth. A comprehensive guide to the administration of entonox is given by Mallett and Bailey (1996).

The entonox cylinder is generally fitted with a Bodok seal connected to a mask or mouthpiece by tubing. It is only operated on active inhalation by the patient; when the patient exhales the gas flow stops. Thus the entonox is delivered on demand. Only properly trained nurses or midwives should administer entonox.

7.8 Route of administration of analgesics

This section covers the salient features of the different routes of drug administration, and outlines some points to consider when selecting appropriate routes of administration.

Oral

The oral route of drug administration is the simplest and for most patients the preferred route. It is the route of administration recommended by the WHO for giving opioids for cancer patients and should be the first choice wherever possible.

Table 7.12 Medication for migraine.

Drug	Oral doses	Side effects	Formulations
Drugs to relieve migraine			
Aspirin	300–900 mg/dose q 4–6 h (maximum 4 g/day)	Nausea and vomiting, indigestion	Tablets, suppositories
Codeine	30–60 mg/day 4–6 times daily (maximum 240 mg/day)	Constipation	Tablets, liquid, injection
Paracetamol	500 mg-1 g/dose q 4–6 h (maximum 4 g/day)	Nausea	Tablets, capsules, liquid, suppositories
Ergotamine	1–2 mg/dose q 30 min (maximum 6 mg/day or 12 mg/week) 6 inhalations/24 h or 15/week	Nausea and vomiting	Tablets, suppositories, inhalation
Sumatriptan	100 mg (maximum 300 mg/24 h) 6 mg subcutaneously (maximum 12 mg/24 h)	Transient sensations of flushing or tingling	Tablets, subcutaneous injection
Drugs to prevent migraine			
Clonidine	50–75 µg 2–3 × daily	Drowsiness, dry mouth, constipation. Can potentiate depression	Tablets, capsules, injection
Methysergide	1–2 mg 2–3 × daily	Nausea, lassitude, weight gain. Risk of retroperitoneal fibrosis – should be given under hospital supervision	Tablets
Pizotifen	0.5–3 mg/day at night or 3 × daily	Increased appetite and weight gain	Tablets, liquid
Propranolol	40 mg 2–3 × daily	Lethargy, cold extremities. Useful in patients with hypertension or anxiety	Tablets, capsules, injection

Compiled from the *BMA Guide to Medicines and Drugs* and *MIMS.*
The manufacturer's SPC (summary of product characteristics) sheet should always be consulted for full prescribing information.

Buccal and sublingual administration

The oral cavity is rich in blood vessels and the absorption of drugs, provided they have appropriate characteristics, is rapid and direct into the systemic circulation. This property can be used to circumvent first-pass metabolism, to produce faster absorption and where local effects in the mouth are desirable.

> First-pass metabolism. Many drugs are metabolised extensively in the liver. Since the vessels draining the stomach and upper intestine pass directly to the liver, via the hepatic portal vein, many absorbed substances are metabolised in the liver before reaching the systemic circulation. If this so-called first-pass metabolism is extensive, then the drug will never appear in useful concentrations in the general circulation.

Glyceryl nitrate is commonly given sublingually, since it is metabolised almost completely by the liver after absorption from the intestine. The formulations available are tablets and an aerosol spray. Administration by this route provides a rapid onset treatment for acute attacks of angina pectoris. Nifedipine may also be given sublingually for acute attacks.

Morphine may be given by tablets which are allowed to dissolve slowly in the mouth (buccal) or under the tongue (sublingual), where they are absorbed by the oral mucosa. Comparisons of oral, the older type of sustained release and buccal administration shows that bioavailability is similar for oral and sustained release preparations (24% and 22% respectively, but lower with the buccal preparation, which is 19%). Buccal preparations also take longer to be absorbed, with time to peak plasma values being 45 minutes for the oral preparation, 2.5 hours for sustained release tablets and 6 hours for the buccal preparation (Hoskin *et al.*, 1989). The newer sustained release preparations show a peak absorption around 7–9 hours after administration. These preparations are useful in patients who have difficulty swallowing tablets and also wish to avoid an injection.

Ergotamine can be given sublingually for migraine where nausea and vomiting preclude the use of tablets.

Intranasal

Very few analgesics are given intranasally, although opioids have been used by this route. A pilot study has been carried out with inhaled fentanyl which suggests that opioids might be successfully administered via this route (Worsley *et al.*, 1990), and intranasal buprenorphine has been used postoperatively.

Rectal

Rectal administration is useful in patients who cannot take oral medication, although some patients are resistant to this route of administration on aesthetic grounds. It is also useful to avoid direct adverse effects of a drug on the stomach or small bowel. Where there is a problem with drug absorption from the stomach, the rectal route may increase the systemic availability of a drug; and since the venous drainage of the rectum avoids the hepatic portal circulation, the rectal route also avoids first-pass metabolism. Drugs can also be given via the rectum where a direct local effect on the rectum and large bowel is desired.

NSAIDs can produce several untoward effects on the stomach and small intestine, and therefore rectal formulations of several of the commonly used NSAIDs have been produced. However, there is no evidence that this route of administration reduces any of these complications (Aronson, 1991).

Drugs for migraine may be given rectally since nausea and vomiting are often part of the condition which prevents absorption of orally administered drugs.

Local anaesthetics for the relief of pain due to haemorrhoids are given by suppository.

The absorption characteristics of opioids given by this route vary widely. Suppository formulations containing morphine, hydromorphone, oxymorphone or oxycodone are available.

It should be noted that drugs are not always evenly distributed throughout a suppository. The practice of cutting a suppository in half to halve the dose is, therefore, not sound. Where this approach really cannot be avoided, the suppository should be cut lengthways, rather than across, as a the majority of the drug is contained at the tip. This cutting also retains the shape of the suppository which is designed to aid insertion.

Transdermal

Some drugs can be absorbed through the skin, and this has given rise to the production of formulations designed to cross the skin and produce effects locally or to be absorbed into the systemic circulation. Transdermal absorption is convenient for the patient and can be used to maintain a constant supply of drug. Transdermal patches are applied to skin, usually on the torso, as the blood supply to the limbs is insufficient, and the drug is absorbed at a constant rate throughout the day and night.

Skin patches containing a depot of fentanyl have been produced. When transdermal opioid preparations are used initially they may need to be supplemented with oral opioid, as the system takes some time to equilibrate. Patches should be replaced every 72 hours, and stable plasma levels are usually achieved by the second dose (Portenoy *et al.*, 1993). Patches may not adhere well to hairy skin or where patients sweat a lot. Patients should be advised to use a new site each time a new patch is applied, but always in the same anatomical region.

Glyceryl trinitrate is given by the transdermal route to avoid first-pass metabolism.

Several NSAIDs are available as creams or ointments. Transdermal absorption provides high concentrations of drug near the site of pain or injury. Since these drugs work by preventing sensitisation of nociceptors, a high concentration locally at the site of inflammation may be especially useful.

Drug delivery systems

A vast range of drug delivery systems is now available to assist in the administration of analgesic agents via the IV, SC, intraspinal and intra-ventricular routes. These systems are more commonly used in the management of acute pain. IV access can be achieved using central catheters, tunnelled catheters and implanted ports (Brandt, 1995). Venous access devices are normally attached to an ambulatory pump which allows for continuous infusion of opioids. The pumps are small and lightweight which means that they do not interfere with patients' ability to carry out their activities of daily living. Infusions provide a constant dose of drug which helps to achieve a constant level of analgesia. In patients who require very large doses of opioids or who already have IV access, a continuous IV infusion may be the most appropriate mode of delivery (Coyle *et al.*, 1995).

The use of venous access devices is not without disadvantages. The catheters require meticulous care in order to prevent infection and mechanical problems can occur with the pumps. This is particularly problematic when the patient is at home. Furthermore, the responsibility of caring for the pump and catheter may cause significant anxiety for patients and families (Whedon & Ferrell, 1991). This highlights the importance of having a member of the healthcare team available around the clock to respond to any problem that may occur with the catheter or pump. The high costs associated with this form of drug delivery also needs to be borne in mind.

Intravenous

The intravenous route provides the most rapid means of delivering analgesia. It is usually opioids that are given by the intravenous route. Methadone will be effective within 2–5 minutes, morphine after 10–15 minutes. It is useful for patients with rapidly escalating pain, or where immediate pain control is required, such as postoperatively. Repeated intravenous injections give a widely fluctuating profile of plasma opioid levels and are therefore not so useful for long-term maintenance, as trough levels in plasma concentration may allow breakthrough pain to occur. Intravenous injections are useful during the initial phase of opioid analgesia and can allow the patient to be made comfortable and give time for dose titration. Intravenous administration avoids first-pass metabolism.

Subcutaneous

If IV access is not available, a subcutaneous infusion offers a suitable alternative, particularly where the patient is at home. An SC infusion can be established by inserting a 27 gauge or similar butterfly needle into a subcutaneous site and attaching a syringe driver. Continuous subcutaneous infusions with battery operated syringe drivers were first used for analgesic administration to deliver diamorphine to patients with advanced cancer. The infusion site can normally be maintained for up to seven days (Breneis *et al.*, 1987). Infusion pumps can be used easily by patients who are at home as the syringe can easily be loaded by a nurse without having to insert a needle. Complications associated with this intervention include redness, leakage and swelling. Pneumothorax following the insertion of a butterfly needle over the ribs has also been reported, and it is recommended that the needle is inserted parallel to the ribs to prevent this complication. Subcutaneous infusions of drugs ranging from chemotherapy agents, analgesics, anti-emetics, anxiolytics and steroids are commonly used and may be particularly welcome for cancer patients in the terminal phase of their illness when they are unable to take oral medication.

Intramuscular

The intramuscular route of injection is useful where there are no personnel available who are trained to give intravenous injections or where rapid treatment is necessary but venous access is difficult. There are a few drugs where the intramuscular route is preferred – for example, when giving adrenaline for an anaphylactic reaction and rapid activity is essential, but when an intravenous injection would cause serious cardiac arrythmias.

The intramuscular route of administration is convenient and takes 30–60 minutes to be effective. Absorption of opioids is variable but repeat dosing can maintain reasonably steady levels of drug. A major drawback is that the injections themselves are painful. Intramuscular injections are contraindicated in patients with haematological malignancy or in those receiving myelotoxic chemotherapy due to risks of bleeding and haematoma formation and the risks of infection.

Several NSAIDs are licensed for intramuscular administration, but these drugs can cause severe local reactions (pain, skin necrosis and abscesses), especially when given into the thigh. Therefore, it might be worth considering a suppository before intramuscular injection.

The usual site of intramuscular injection is the anterolateral aspect of the mid-thigh, although there are some exceptions, such as NSAIDs where the gluteal muscles are recommended. The skin should be drawn back before injection as injection is easier through tight skin. Once the needle has been inserted the plunger should be drawn back and held for 5 seconds to ensure that the needle tip is not in a blood vessel. Releasing the tension on the skin after injection causes the needle track through the muscle and subcutaneous fat to be separated, and thus the risk of back-leakage is reduced (Aronson, 1995).

Spinal

Spinal opioids have been used extensively in the management of intractable severe pain. Morphine is the usual opioid used, others are fentanyl or pethidine. Only solutions formulated for spinal administration must be used, as some other formulations may contain potentially neurotoxic preservatives.

In cancer patients the spinal route is only used for those who experience excessive side effects or intractable pain when opioids are administered via the oral, IV, SC or transdermal route, although spinal opioids have been shown to produce profound analgesia with lower doses than would be needed for other routes of administration (Plummer *et al.*, 1991).

Spinal means administration of the opioid close to the spinal cord; it can be given by epidural, intrathecal or subarachnoid administration. All routes can be accessed using temporary or permanent catheters or an implanted port. Introducing the opioid close to the spinal cord results in a much higher concentration of opioid at spinal receptors, and hence a greater degree of pain relief, than would be achieved by systemic administration. Stimulation of spinal receptors is an important component of pain control. Opioid receptors both pre-synaptically and post-synaptically prevent transmission of nociceptive inputs from primary afferent neurones (see Chapter 2). Opioid receptors in the brain will also be reached by opioids given spinally due to the cephalad (towards the head) migration of cerebro-spinal fluid (CSF) (Gourlay *et al.*, 1985) contributing to both analgesia and side effects. Vascular uptake from the CSF also results in significant plasma concentration of opioid.

The intraspinal route of opioid administration has been widely used for the management of postoperative pain, especially after thoracic, orthopaedic and major abdominal surgery and following caesarean section (Joint College of Surgeons and Anaesthetists, 1990).

Side effects of spinally administered opioids can be well controlled and are generally less common in patients previously treated with systemic opioids. Urinary retention and puritis are more common with the intraspinal than with the oral or parenteral routes. Low blood pressure is not a problem with intraspinal opioids but can be problematic when anaesthetics are given by this route. A somewhat curious side effect of spinal opioids is that they cause itching, occurring in up to 46% of patients receiving spinal drug (Ballantyne *et al.*, 1988). The itch may be general, have a segmental distribution or be localised to the nose and face.

In general spinal administration is employed where systemic opioids fail to provide adequate analgesia and/or are associated with unacceptable side effects. Spinal administration avoids sympathetic blockade and postural hypotension, but marked sedation can occur if higher doses are used, along with the other commonly observed side effects of opioids.

The best response to spinal opioids is obtained in patients with deep, constant somatic pain. Patients with cancer pain have variable responses. Spinal opioids have been successful in cases of neuropathic and deafferentation pain (Plummer *et al.*, 1991).

Spinal opioids may be given as single injections or continuous infusions. Epidural administration requires a surgical operation to implant a cannula in the epidural space and connect this to a reservoir. It is, therefore, not widely used and is employed mainly in the palliative setting where other routes of administration are not possible. Skilled professional support needs to be available to ensure that the system works well and does not place too much of a burden on patients and their relatives.

Patient controlled analgesia (PCA)

Patient controlled analgesia refers to a system where the patient self-administers analgesic drugs, thus titrating their medication to their pain experience. This can be achieved with oral medication, but the term PCA is more commonly used to describe the use of a specially designed infusion pump which can deliver a bolus of analgesic via the IV, SC or intraspinal route on demand. These pumps were initially adopted into the management of postsurgical pain. By setting a 'lockout' period when the equipment is unresponsive for a certain period after each dose, a maximum limit is put on the amount of drug which could be given in any 24-hour period. Patients could then administer their own analgesic drugs as required.

PCA increased in popularity for patients with long-term pain (such as cancer patients) when devices were developed which allowed a combination of continuous infusion and demand dosing to be delivered by the same piece of equipment. Patients may now have a constant maintenance dose of opioid by infusion which can be 'topped-up' by the patient when breakthrough pain occurs (see Lindley, 1994, for review).

The advantage of PCA lies in its flexibility, lack of delay in administration and the fact that patients are provided with some degree of control over their situation. PCA has been shown to reduce significantly the dosage of opioids, to provide a more consistent level of analgesia, to save nursing time and facilitate earlier discharge from hospital following surgery (Joint College of Surgeons and Anaesthetists, 1990; Inturissi, 1992; Koh & Thomas, 1994). Psychological factors are thought to play a large part in patients' acceptance and use of PCA (Thomas & Rose, 1993). A comprehensive review of PCA can be found in Heath and Thomas' book (1993).

The main advantages and disadvantages of the different routes of administration of analgesics are summarised in Table 7.13.

7.9 Surgical techniques for pain control

If the source of pain can be identified as mechanical – for example, compression of a nerve or distension of an organ – surgical interventions may be appropriate. These interventions consist of mobilising tissue to relieve tension or by reinforcing collagenous tissue. In cancer patients, or those presenting with benign tumours, surgery may involve removing the tumour mass.

Conservative methods may be recommended for pain of mechanical origin, which should respond to rest and removal of the mechanical insult.

Where pain relief cannot be obtained by drugs or by non-invasive procedures such as physiotherapy, the application of heat or cold, or complementary therapy, then it may be decided to employ surgical techniques to interrupt nerve pathways. Since these are fairly invasive procedures, they are not the first line of treatment. These techniques are considered below.

Blocking transmission of noxious stimuli

The transmission of noxious stimuli can be blocked by stopping transmission, either temporarily or permanently, in the peripheral or central nervous system. This can be achieved by

- agents which act at the level of pain receptors, such as NSAIDs;
- techniques which block peripheral axonal transmission such as local anaesthetic agents injected into the appropriate nerve or neurolytic blockade;
- spinal or epidural block by drugs or neurolytic techniques;
- blockade of sympathetic ganglion function by local anaesthetics or neurolytic blockade.

Neurolytic – neuro = nerve; lysis = fragmenting, breaking or destroying. Hence, an agent which destroys nerves.

The action of NSAIDs has been covered above.

Table 7.13 Main advantages and disadvantages of common routes of opioid administration.

Route	Advantages	Disadvantages
Oral	Effective for both localised and generalised pain Multiple drug choice Can be administered by patient, family or carers Some inexpensive Sustained release opioids available Rapid onset of action for angina	Side effects (nausea and vomiting) may limit use Patient condition (profound weakness, swallowing difficulties) may limit use
Transdermal opioids (Fentanyl)	Long duration of action (48–73 h) Allow strong opioid to be used in outpatient setting Useful for patients intolerant to morphine Easy to use Continuous opioid without needles or pumps Can be administered by patient, family or carers	Side effects may not be quickly reversible Difficult to modify dose rapidly Slow onset of action Require rescue medication for breakthrough pain Do not stick to hairy or sweaty skin Expensive
Rectal	Relatively easy-to-use alternative when oral route not possible Can be administered by patient or family Alternative opioids available for morphine intolerant patients Less expensive and more convenient than subcutaneous or intravenous	Not universally accepted Side effects of opioids may limit analgesic effectiveness Relatively slow onset of action Contraindicated if low white cell count (risk of infection, bleeding)

Route		
Subcutaneous	Can provide rapid pain relief without intravenous access Morphine and diamorphine are preferred opioids for this route When used as PCA allows for rapid dose titration and provides patient with sense of control	Only limited volume can be infused (usually 2–4 ml/hour) Induration and irritation at infusion site may be a complication Requires skilled nursing and pharmacy support Expensive drug infusion pump required Costs of disposables
Intravenous	Can provide rapid pain relief Most opioids can be given by this route Not limited by volume When used as PCA allows rapid dose titration and gives patient sense of control	Infection and infiltration of iv lines are potential complications Requires skilled nursing and pharmacy support Often requires expensive pumps Costs of disposables
Spinal (epidural or intrathecal)	Useful for pain relief that has not responded to less invasive measures Local anaesthetics may be added to the opioid to increase analgesia	Tolerance may occur sooner than with oral or rectal administration Infection at catheter site can occur Pruritis and urinary retention more common with this route Contraindicated in presence of spinal cord compression Requires special expertise Requires special monitoring May require expensive drug infusion pumps. Costs of disposables

Modified from *Agency for Health Care Policy and Research (AHCPR) Handbook.*

Peripheral anaesthetics and neurolytic blockade

Temporary blockade of neuronal transmission can be achieved by injecting local anaesthetics in the region of the appropriate nerve. More permanent destruction of peripheral nerves may be achieved by coagulating the nerve with cold (cryocoagulation) or by radiofrequency coagulation. Neurolytic agents such as ethanol (ethyl alcohol) or phenol can also be used.

In general, neurolytic blocks are best suited to patients with short life expectancy who suffer from well-localised pain that has proven difficult to control with other measures, since there are complications with these techniques. The main problems are that denervation is a stimulus for nerves to repair or regrow. Re-innervation occurs about 6 weeks after cryocoagulation and 12 months following radiofrequency coagulation (Bogduk, 1989). The denervation may also produce deafferentation pain, and incomplete neural destruction may produce a neuralgic type of pain (Swarm & Cousins, 1993). Both of these problems may be treated by transcutaneous electrical nerve stimulation (TENS) or centrally acting drugs.

The problem of regeneration pain occurs because nerve coagulation leaves cell bodies intact. Destruction of the dorsal root ganglia may give a more permanent pain relief. Such ganglionolysis too has its problems in that it can produce numbness and or denervation hypersensitivity.

A ganglion is a collection of nerve cell bodies. The axons arising from the cell bodies form a nerve. The dorsal root ganglions are the cell bodies of the primary nociceptive afferents (see Chapter 2).

Spinal blockade

Blocking the transmission of nociceptive information in the spinal cord may be achieved by spinal administration of opioid drugs or by surgical destruction of a small region of the spinal pathway. The spinal administration of opioids has been covered above.

Neurolytic spinal techniques

A more permanent blockade of spinal pathways is produced by injection of phenol or alcohol close to the spine. Neurolytic agents may be given into the subarachnoid, epidural or subdural spaces.

- Spinal – all routes of administration near or within the spinal cord;
- Epidural – immediately outside the dura mater, within the spinal vertebral canal;
- Intrathecal – inside the thecal sac or dura mater (includes the subdural space);
- Subdural – between the dura mater and arachnoid mater;
- Subarachnoid – inside the arachnoid mater, into the CSF.

The subdural space is wider at the cervical region and this route is easier to use for blocking nerves which serve the cervical, head and neck region. This includes treating pain in ears, nose and throat.

The epidural route is used to access and block nerves supplying the neck, shoulders and arms. Subarachnoid blockade is used for lower parts of the body, such as pain associated with colostomy, colon cancer and permanent bladder catheters.

All these techniques are used to produce local destruction of nerves, so they should be restricted to situations where the pain field relates to one or two spinal segments. The techniques are not so effective for widely disseminated pain.

Percutaneous cordotomy

Severe pain in the lower body can be treated by cordotomy. This involves interrupting the ascending spino-thalamic tract by sectioning the nerves of this tract. Sensation is lost on the opposite side of the body (remember the nerves contributing to the spino-thalamic tract cross the spinal cord in the anterior commissure) and sensation will be lost in nerves that enter the cord above the section and for a few segments below the section.

Neurolytic sympathetic blockade

Sympathetically maintained pain can also be treated by neurolytic block of sympathetic nerves. Neurolytic sympathetic blockade offers the greatest relief for patients with visceral pain. Patients with mixed somatic–visceral pain are likely to have incomplete pain relief following sympathetic blockade. Severe combined somatic and visceral pain is best managed by techniques such as spinal opioids; but the two techniques may be used in conjunction where the sympathetic blockade helps to reduce the dose of spinal opioid needed.

Chemical or surgical lumbar sympathectomy

Chemical or surgical lumbar sympathectomy may be used to relieve pain due to vascular disease. Ischaemia and cellulitis can cause severe pain in patients with inoperable peripheral vascular disease. This pain may cause increased sympathetic discharge, sensitising nociceptors and setting up a vicious circle of sympathetically maintained pain (see Chapter 2). Lumbar sympathectomy blocks the sympathetic efferent fibres that control vascular tone in the lower half of the body. It has been shown to reduce ischaemic rest pain, increase blood flow and enhance healing of the chronic ulcers that can occur in this condition.

Pain due to pelvic cancers responds to this technique. If there is extensive pelvic and abdominal spread of malignant disease, a combination of coeliac plexus and lumbar sympathetic blocks may be needed.

7.10 Radiotherapy for pain control

As well as being used for the treatment of cancer, radiotherapy has an important role in palliative care of cancer patients. Tumour mass may be contained by radiotherapy treatment, and external radiobeam therapy is a standard treatment for painful bony metastases. This is associated with few side effects. Where bony metastases are widespread, hemibody or total-body irradiation may be necessary.

Radionuclides for bony metastases

Total-body or hemibody irradiation, while successful for treating bone pain, has the disadvantage of multiple side effects since all the tissue in the irradiated area will receive the same dose of radiation. The most problematic of these are immunosupression, gastro-intestinal problems and radiation pneumonitis. In an attempt to avoid these problems a technique has been developed whereby radioactive bone seeking compounds are given to the patient. The radiopharmaceutical deposits in bone and emits low-dose radiation, usually beta radiation, locally to control bone pain. Rhenium-186-1,1-hydroxyethylidine diphosphonate has been evaluated in a number of small-scale studies where initial results show effective palliation of bone pain from breast or prostate metastases (Maxon *et al.*, 1991). Phosphorus-32 and strontium-89 are radioisotopes that have been in use for bone pain for several decades, but their use dwindled after the introduction of external beam therapy. Recently, strontium-89 has been re-evaluated for use in bony metastases where it too is proving effective in control of bone pain.

7.11 Stimulation of descending pathways

The endogenous analgesic pathways can be stimulated within the CNS. These neuroaugmentative procedures employ electrodes and pulse generators similar to pacemaker systems. The electrodes must be implanted in cortical, brain-stem or spinal regions. Percutaneous spinal cord stimulation has proved useful in different types of pain, although experience in cancer pain is limited (Lamer, 1994).

Small series of patients have received deep-brain stimulation from electrodes implanted stereotaxically in the periaqueductal grey matter, the periventricular grey or the thalamic area. Such techniques are currently only available at specialist centres and are likely to be employed for severe cases, or where other, less-invasive procedures have failed. Complications include infection, haemorrhage, and diplopia (double vision) (Lamer, 1994).

Summary of Chapter 7

- Opioids remain the cornerstone of treatment of severe pain, yet there are many reservations to using them.
- The WHO Three Step Ladder is a useful paradigm to help with selection of appropriate analgesia.
- Opioids come in a variety of formulations and can be administered by different routes.
- The mechanism of action of opioids and the main drugs in this class are reviewed.
- Adjuvant drugs are drugs which may have a different primary indication but can be used alone or in combination with other analgesics to control pain.
- NSAIDs are a large class of useful analgesics which also have anti-pyretic and anti-inflammatory properties.
- Specific conditions (e.g. migraine, angina) require specific drugs for control. These are discussed.
- The routes by which analgesics may be administered is reviewed and the possible advantages of different routes summarised.
- In cases of severe or intractable pain, surgery may be the only resort. The common analgesic surgical techniques are outlined.

Chapter 8

Treatment of Pain: Complementary and Non-invasive Techniques

It is repeatedly emphasised in the literature (and in this book) that pain is not the result of a single physiological or pharmacological event, and it has been discussed in detail how pain is an experience that encompasses the whole individual. Many factors of personality, upbringing, the meaning and the circumstances of the pain interact to produce the overall pain experience. So, it is not surprising that pain responds to a variety of different treatments and often only a combination of different treatments will give total pain control. This chapter discusses the non-invasive, complementary interventions that are used in the battle against pain.

8.1 Cognitive-behavioural strategies

In recent years cognitive-behavioural strategies have emerged as effective non-pharmacological interventions for the management of different types of pain. These strategies are particularly useful in situations where psychosocial factors are contributing significantly to the patient's pain experience. The goal of cognitive-behavioural interventions is to decrease pain perception as opposed to making the pain disappear. This is achieved as a result of patients acquiring a range of cognitive and behavioural coping skills which provide them with a greater sense of control over their pain (Fishman & Loscalzo, 1987; Turk & Meichenbaum, 1994; Arathuzik, 1994). Cognitive-behavioural strategies range in complexity from simple distraction to more complicated interventions such as systematic desensitisation and hypnosis (Table 8.1).

Cognitive-behavioural strategies

Cognitive-behavioural strategies include a range of different interventions which are aimed at changing the patient's perception of pain, altering dysfunctional pain behaviours and fostering a sense of control over pain.

Table 8.1 Cognitive-behavioural strategies.

- Distraction
- Focusing
- Reframing
- Music therapy
- Guided imagery
- Relaxation
- Biofeedback
- Hypnosis
- Systematic desensitisation

Distraction

Essentially distraction is all about taking patients' minds off their pain. When patients use distraction they focus their attention on a stimulus other than their pain, thereby banishing the pain to the periphery of their awareness (McCaffrey, 1990). There are three different types of distraction which can be used in the management of pain (Fishman & Loscalzo, 1987). First, imaginative inattention, a strategy where one would imagine oneself doing something very pleasant such as walking in the forest, going on a family outing or floating on water. Second, mental distraction where the person carries out some mental activity such as counting, reciting a poem, or praying. Finally, behavioural task distraction is a strategy where the person actually does something that they find to be pleasant such as watching television, listening or watching a humorous audio or video tape, petting an animal, reading a book, smelling an essential oil or talking with friends.

Many patients will have worked out for themselves effective ways of distracting their attention from their pain. These strategies, which are often very idiosyncratic, may have been used by patients with great success for many years. Copp (1974; 1990) found that some hospitalised patients felt inhibited about using their usual pain coping behaviours because they might be 'against the rules' of the hospital or be laughed at by healthcare professionals because they were not scientific. This emphasises the importance of discovering what patients normally do to control their pain and encouraging them to incorporate these strategies into their plan of care. This does not preclude the use of other distraction techniques. The nurse should work with the patient to create innovative distraction methods that are limited '... only by the creativity of the nurse in combination with the creativity, abilities and preferences of the patient.' (Mobily *et al.*, 1993).

Distraction is particularly useful in the management of pain related to procedures such as dressing changes or lumbar punctures. McCaffrey and Beebe (1994) have outlined the following characteristics of effective distraction strategies for brief episodes of pain:

- Interesting to the patient.
- Consistent with the patient's energy level and ability to concentrate.
- Rhythm should be included and emphasised, e.g. keeping time to music.
- Stimulates the major sensory modalities: hearing, vision, touch, smell, movement.
- Capable of providing a change in stimuli when the pain changes, e.g. increased stimuli for increased pain.

There are a few points which need to be remembered when facilitating a patient to use distraction. First, rehearse the distraction technique with the patient prior to the painful procedure. Second, commence the distraction before the patient begins to experience pain. Finally, remember that distraction alone may not be enough to prevent or alleviate pain; other interventions may be required.

It seems important at this stage to reiterate a point made in Chapter 5. When patients are using distraction as a means to control their pain it is very easy for healthcare professionals to misinterpret this behaviour as an indication that the patient is not in pain. The onus is on the professional to ensure that a proper assessment is carried out and that assumptions are not made about the patient's level of pain. It is also important to remember that after patients have stopped using distraction they may experience increased awareness of pain, and an increase in fatigue and irritability (McCaffrey & Beebe, 1994). Other interventions should be offered at this stage to prevent the pain worsening.

Music therapy

Music has been used with great success to distract patients' attention away from their pain. According to Larsen Beck (1991) there are a number of possible mechanisms by which music can ameliorate pain including distraction, increased relaxation, reduction in anxiety, counterstimulation and increased feelings of control. The most effective type of music at decreasing anxiety and inducing relaxation is music with a slow steady rhythm and low frequency tones. However, some patients may find that fast lively music mobilises energy which in turn helps them to cope more effectively with their pain (McCaffrey, 1990).

A range of different types of music should be available so that patients are able to choose the type of music which is most preferable and relaxing for them. For this reason the use of a cassette tape or CD is better than the radio. Headphones should be used to cut down on outside noises and to avoid disturbing other people. Some patients will find it helpful to adjust the volume according to the level of their pain or to tap out the rhythm of the music. Both of these activities will help increase the patient's concentration on the distraction. Music has been shown to be effective at ameliorating pain across a number of treatment settings including post-operative (Locsin, 1981), oncology (Zimmerman *et al.*, 1989; Larsen Beck, 1991), coronary care, during childbirth (Cianciolo Livingston, 1985), with children (Ryan, 1989) and during nursing procedures (Angus & Faux, 1989).

Focusing

Focusing consists of a number of cognitive coping techniques which are quite different from those used in distraction (Fishman and Loscalzo, 1987). The first strategy is imaginative transformation where one imagines one's pain as an entity which can be controlled. An example would be viewing one's pain as heat radiating from an oven and then imagining that it can be controlled by turning the oven off. The second is imaginative transformation of context where one imagines a different context and therefore meaning for one's pain. An example would be imagining oneself as an injured football player during a cup final continuing to play in order to win the game. The final strategy is dissociated somatisation where one would imagine the painful body part as not being part of oneself.

Reframing

Reframing, otherwise known as cognitive modification, helps patients to identify and correct distorted perceptions, misinterpretations, unrealistic expectations, and irrational beliefs about pain (Fishman & Loscalzo, 1987). Essentially the patient is taught to replace negative thoughts and beliefs with more positive ones. This approach is particularly useful for patients with chronic pain who often experience feelings of helplessness and hopelessness and have a tendency to personalise and dramatise negative life events (Slater & Good, 1991). Fishman and Loscalzo (1987) have outlined the process of cognitive modification as follows:

1. Identify dysfunctional automatic thoughts and images (cognitions) as they pass through consciousness and learn to monitor them.
2. Recognise the specific connection between the occurrences of emotions and behaviours and the types of automatic thoughts or images that precede or accompany them.
3. Substitute more functional (reasonable) thoughts or images (cognitions) for the identified dysfunctional thoughts.
4. Identify and alter dysfunctional underlying beliefs and attitudes.
5. Practice coping and modification techniques.

Relaxation

There is a lot of evidence available which demonstrates the relationship between pain, muscle tension, autonomic hyperarousal and anxiety, and therefore it makes sense to use an intervention which causes a relaxation response when trying to ameliorate pain. A variety of different techniques have been designed to bring about a state of physical and mental relaxation (Table 8.2). These techniques are often used in combination with guided imagery and biofeedback.

Table 8.2   Techniques which induce a relaxation response.

- Deep breathing exercises
- Passive relaxation
- Jaw relaxation
- Progressive muscle relaxation
- Meditation
- Autogenic training
- Hypnosis

Some relaxation techniques are very brief and simple to use, for example, yawning or deep breathing exercises; others are much more time consuming and complicated. Passive relaxation is where the person focuses their attention, in a systematic fashion, on sensations of warmth in various parts of the body and on how the tension is dissipating in these areas (Fishman & Loscalzo, 1987). Progressive muscle relaxation, one of the most commonly used relaxation techniques, is a process of systematically focusing attention on various muscle groups in the body. The person is encouraged to tense and then to release the tension from a particular muscle group and then to move on to the next muscle group in a stepwise fashion (Sloman, 1995). Meditation is where the person mentally chants a word or sentence which in turn helps to draw their attention away from their distressing experience and to induce a relaxed state.

Hypnosis is a very sophisticated and complex way of bringing about the relaxation response, and therefore, it is administered by a trained therapist. This therapist can teach a patient to self-administer hypnosis. When hypnotised, a person is in a state of deep relaxation and is very receptive to suggestions. Hypnosis is used to promote relaxation, to decrease negative emotions and to help patients shift their attention away from their pain (Fishman & Loscalzo, 1987). The efficacy of hypnosis has been established for a number of different pain syndromes including labour pain, cancer pain, postoperative pain, dental pain, and for migraine and other types of headaches (Spiegal & Bloom, 1983).

Relaxation therapies need to be used with caution in patients with bradycardia, heart block or hypotension since there is a danger that the physiologic effects which accompany the relaxation response may exacerbate their condition. This is an important consideration in the immediate postoperative period when the patient may be also given intravenous morphine to ameliorate pain (see Chapter 6). There is also a theoretical risk that relaxation may result in adverse psychological effects in psychotic patients (Spross & Wolff Burke, 1995). Levin *et al.* (1987) point out that any technique which involves tensing of muscles may exacerbate postoperative discomfort. For this reason it is probably prudent to avoid the use of progressive muscle relaxation in the post-operative setting. Moreover, this technique should not be used in patients who are prone to muscle cramps or spasms and may not be useful in frail or confused elderly patients.

Guided imagery

Guided imagery is a cognitive technique which involves using one's mind to create or experience a mental image which in turn either distracts attention away from the pain experience or focuses attention directly on to the pain. Any one or all of the senses can be used to create these pictures. If patients want to direct attention away from the pain they are encouraged to imagine they are somewhere pleasant and relaxing. For example, a person may imagine that they are walking bare-foot in a forest. They can feel the coolness of the forest floor on their feet, and hear the breeze rustle the leaves on the trees. They can smell wild flowers and see all the beauty around them.

Alternatively, patients may focus directly on their pain by imagining that they are fighting or controlling it in some way. For example, they could visualise their pain as a dragon and then imagine themselves slaying the dragon. Such an image can provide patients with a real sense of control over their pain experience which may contribute to a reduction in anxiety and an increased state of relaxation.

Guided imagery can be self-guided or other-guided. Many patients may find the other-guided approach easier when first learning to use guided imagery. As they become used to the technique they can start to use the self-guided approach. It is best to ask patients to identify their own evocative images as opposed to using a standard scenario, as some images can be very unpleasant for the patient. Some of the focusing and reframing techniques mentioned earlier on in this chapter can be used as part of a guided imagery intervention.

Guided imagery may result in some patients becoming more anxious and upset because it can open a door to unresolved emotional issues. This can have both positive and negative effects. It can be positive in that the unresolved emotions may be contributing to the pain experience (see Chapter 4) and imagery may be a potent way of releasing these emotions (Kearney, 1996). If these emotions can be dealt with successfully, the person's pain may be ameliorated. Alternatively, the release of emotions may be too much for a person to bear or deal with at a particular moment in time and the imagery will have only succeeded in raising anxiety and distress with no positive effects. Relaxation exercises are often used in conjunction with guided imagery and these may enhance the effect of the imagery (Sofaer, 1992).

Biofeedback

Biofeedback is a technique where the person receives some form of auditory or visual signal which indicates some change in a biological process (Jessop & Gallegos, 1994). This signal is intended to increase awareness of how the person is responding in different situations. The goal of biofeedback is to help the person to learn how to relax chronically tensed muscles or chronically aroused autonomic functions.

Feedback can be received about the amount of electricity generated by a muscle or muscle group (electromyogram (EMG)), skin temperature, skin resistance, pulse, blood pressure, and waveforms of the electro-encephalogram (EEG). This technique can be applied using complex technologies such as a biofeedback machine or very simply by counting a pulse. It should be remembered, however, that biofeedback is not used in a vacuum, some other intervention such as counselling or relaxation training is also employed. Biofeedback has been used to help ameliorate pain across a wide spectrum of pain syndromes such as muscle contraction headaches, migraine, back pain and labour pain, with varied degrees of success. Readers are referred to the work by Jessop and Gallegos (1994) for a more extensive review on biofeedback.

8.2 Cutaneous stimulation

Cutaneous stimulation includes a range of strategies (Table 8.3) which are thought to either increase the transmission of non-noxious inputs into the spinal cord or modulate the transmission of noxious inputs. For example, massage is thought to stimulate large unmyelinated fibres which in turn suppresses the transmission of C-fibre input (see Chapter 2). Interestingly, cutaneous stimulation strategies can be effective when applied to sites other than the site of the pain. These sites include acupuncture or trigger points, and sites proximal, distal or contralateral to the site of the pain (McCaffrey, 1990).

Table 8.3 Cutaneous stimulation strategies.

- Massage
- Vibration
- Application of heat and cold
- Transcutaneous Electrical Nerve Stimulation (TENS)

Cutaneous stimulation

Cutaneous stimulation includes a range of non-invasive methods which are thought to either increase transmission of non-noxious inputs into the spinal cord or modulate the transmission of noxious inputs, both of which result in varying degrees of pain control.

Massage

Massage has been defined as 'stimulation of the skin and underlying tissues with varying degrees of hand pressure to decrease pain, produce relaxation and/or improve circulation' (Mobily *et al.*, 1994). It has been used as a therapeutic intervention for thousands of years. A number of different techniques are employed in massage including stroking or effleurage, connective tissue massage, kneading and petrissage, and friction and deep massage (Haldeman, 1994). Unperfumed lotions, oils or powders are normally used to reduce friction. As well as its direct physiological effect on pain, massage is thought to decrease pain by reducing muscle spasm and tension, improving superficial circulation and reducing oedema. Some people view massage as a powerful means of communicating feelings such as compassion, empathy and caring which may be more effective than verbal communication alone. Indeed, massage may act like a key which opens up avenues of communication which were previously closed. In addition, carers can be taught simple massage techniques. This can help overcome feelings of helplessness and impotence which carers often feel when caring for a seriously ill relative or friend.

When deciding whether to use massage, its benefits must be weighed against how acceptable touch is to a particular patient. Massage may engender huge anxiety and discomfort in those patients who dislike physical touch. On the other hand, the fact that massage is a therapeutic intervention with clearly defined boundaries, may make it acceptable for these patients (McNamara, 1994).

Massage is contraindicated in patients with the following conditions:

- extensive burns;
- deep venous thrombosis and thrombophlebitis;
- extremes of body temperature;
- acute, undiagnosed back pain;
- contagious diseases;
- unstable pregnancy;
- bleeding disorders;
- areas of open lesions and tender skin (Horrigan, 1995).

In addition, massage could be misinterpreted by some as a sexual advance, which could create an embarrassing and awkward situation for the masseur(se) (Spross & Wolff Burke, 1995). Some people have voiced concern over using massage for people with cancer. This concern is based on the belief that massage may encourage the spread of cancer (McNamara, 1994). There is no evidence to support this belief and therefore, it could be argued that the beneficial effects of massage far outweigh the nebulous risk of spreading cancer, although it probably is not wise to massage directly over a palpable tumour. Nor is it advocated to massage areas currently undergoing radiotherapy.

Although massage has been utilised to ameliorate pain for centuries, there is limited scientific evidence to support its use. In recent years a number of nurse researchers have attempted to address this situation. Sims (1986) found that there was a slight but non-significant decrease in subjective reports of pain in six women with breast cancer following massage. In an experimental pilot study of 28 cancer patients, Weinrich and Weinrich (1990) demonstrated a significant decrease in pain in the male subjects in the experimental group following a 10-minute Swedish back massage. Ferrell-Torry and Glick (1993) administered a 30-minute massage consisting of effleurage and petrissage to the feet, back, neck and shoulders of nine male cancer patients. Myofacial trigger point therapy was also administered. They found a significant reduction in mean pain and anxiety scores and an increase in relaxation following the massage. Davies and Riches (1995) administered a 30-minute Swedish back massage to five women with rheumatoid arthritis. Overall the women felt that the massage made them feel better and more relaxed, although only one felt that the massage had any specific effect on her arthritis.

All of these studies are limited by small sample sizes and by the fact that the majority did not employ an experimental design. Despite these limitations, there is evidence to demonstrate the benefits of massage on pain and nurses should consider its use in their every day clinical practice.

Aromatherapy

Aromatherapy is the use of aromatic essential oils to bring about a range of beneficial therapeutic effects. The oils can be used in a number of different ways, including massage, aromatic baths, vaporisation and as hot compresses (Percival, 1995). When using aromatherapy massage the essential oil must be mixed with a carrier oil, such as grapeseed oil, before it is applied to the skin. A number of essential oils are thought to have analgesic and anti-inflammatory properties (Table 8.4). An aromatherapist will choose a combination of oils depending on the patient's needs. Aromatherapy has been advocated to ameliorate back pain, arthritic joint pain, aching muscles and muscle cramps. Great care should be exercised when using essential oils, particularly in very ill patients and young children (McNamara, 1994). There are many poor quality oils in

Table 8.4 Essential oils with analgesic, antispasmodic and anti-inflammatory properties.

- Lavender*
- Chamomile (Roman)*
- Rosemary
- Ginger
- Myrrh
- Bergamot

* Also has sedative and relaxant properties.
Source: Percival (1995).

general circulation which may do more harm than good. It is best to seek the advise of a trained aromatherapist before using aromatherapy.

Despite its growth in popularity amongst nurses, there is limited scientific evidence available to support the use of aromatherapy in clinical practice. Hewitt (1992) found that patients in an intensive care unit benefited from a 20-minute foot massage with lavender oil. The massage led to a marked reduction in heart rate, respiratory rate, blood pressure, pain and wakefulness in comparison to those patients who received massage alone or undisturbed bed rest. A randomised clinical trial (n=635) comparing the use of pure lavender oil, synthetic lavender oil and an inert substance as a bath additive for 10 days following normal childbirth found no statistically significant differences between the groups (Dale & Cornwell, 1994). Nevertheless, this study did show a lower mean discomfort score between day three and five in those women using pure lavender oil and most of the women found using the oil to be a pleasurable experience.

Superficial heat and cold applications

Superficial heat and cold applications offer health professionals a simple and cost-effective non-pharmacological intervention for pain. Many patients will use these applications as a matter of course without any consultation with their caregivers.

Superficial application of heat increases the blood flow to skin and superficial organs which will improve tissue oxygenation and nutrition and aids in the elimination of pain causing substances. Heat can also relax muscle spasm and decrease joint stiffness (Mobily *et al.*, 1994). Heat can be applied in a number of different ways including hot water bottles, hot packs, paraffin baths, moist air, hot and moist compresses, electric heating pads and hot baths. A towel should be wrapped around the heating device to prevent burning and patients should be discouraged from lying directly on the heating device.

A certain amount of controversy exists about the use of superficial heat in cancer patients. Some people express concern that the use of superficial heat in the vicinity of a tumour may facilitate tumour growth and metastatic spread. The scientific evidence to support this viewpoint is extremely limited and therefore, the use of superficial heat as a method of pain control in cancer patients can still be recommended (Jacox *et al.*, 1994). However, it must be emphasised that the use of strategies to deliver deep heat, which are usually administered by physiotherapists, should not be applied directly over a tumour mass.

The superficial application of cold causes vasoconstriction of the skin blood vessels which helps to prevent or reduce swelling following injury and can also decrease the production of pain causing metabolites and conduction in pain fibres (Ernst & Fialka, 1994). Cold application can reduce muscle spasm, decrease muscle tone and spasticity and joint stiffness. It has also been used with success to ameliorate the pain associated with injections (Ross & Soltes, 1995). As with heat applications, cold can be applied in a number of different ways including application of an ice pack, wrapping the affected area with a towel dipped in ice water, ice massage, use of ethylchloride spray, immersion of affected area in ice water and application of a frozen pack of vegetables. With the exception of ice massage, care should be taken to protect the patient's skin from direct exposure to the cold application.

Cold is thought to be more effective, has a shorter duration of application, works quicker and produces a longer lasting effect than heat. Unfortunately, many people are averse to using cold and find heat much more acceptable (McCaffrey, 1990). A cold application can be made more acceptable by adding layers of towel to the ice pack and gradually removing them as the patient becomes accustomed to the cold sensation. Cold should not be used in patients with any condition in which vasoconstriction increases symptoms, such as with Raynaud's syndrome and peripheral vascular disease.

The efficacy of cold and heat applications can be improved by using them interchangeably. There is no set interval for alternating the heat or cold; patients should be encouraged to identify what works best for them. Great care should be exercised when using either heat or cold applications, particularly in patients who are unable to communicate or have decreased or absent sensations. Both applications are also contraindicated in areas which have been previously treated with radiotherapy.

8.3 Therapeutic touch

Therapeutic touch (TT) is rooted on the ancient practice of laying on of hands, a practice which was recorded by the earliest literate cultures

(Krieger, 1975). A number of assumptions underpin the concept of TT: humans are energy fields; there is a close interconnection both between and within humans and their environment; healthy individuals have an excess of energy (also known as prana or Ch'i) which flows in a balanced and synchronised manner; and a blockage or disruption of energy flow or a deficit in energy can result in physical or psychological ill health (Krieger, 1975; Boguslawski, 1980; Owens & Ehrenreich, 1991a).

This view of man as an energy system is well accepted by Eastern philosophies, yet is regarded with much scepticism by Western science. One of the reasons for this is that there is dearth of scientific evidence to explain adequately the phenomenon of human energy fields. TT is used to treat any imbalance in an individual's energy field. This is achieved by a transfer of energy from a healer to the patient and/or a realignment of the patient's energy field (Husband, 1988). The healer must make a conscious attempt to help the subject. This motivation appears to be a significant determinant of the success or otherwise of TT. It is important to point out that the healer's hands can remain about two or three inches from the patient's body. Direct body contact does not need to take place for healing to occur.

The evidence supporting the use of TT in the management of pain is sparse. A small randomised study by Keller and Bzdek (1986) found that TT resulted in a significant reduction in tension headache pain when compared to placebo touch. Although, the literature contains a number of case studies which report the effect of TT (Owens & Ehrenreich, 1991a; Heidt, 1991), such studies do not demonstrate cause and effect relationships in a scientifically rigorous manner, which leads critics of TT to suggest that its efficacy is purely as a result of a placebo effect. Advocates would argue that TT does no harm, has potential benefits and therefore, if the patient is willing to undergo the procedure there is no reason why it should not be used until evidence is produced to the contrary. Conversely, Husband (1988) would caution that you can do a patient a disservice by using TT to just control a symptom, without addressing the cause of the symptom. This viewpoint is supported by Boguslawski (1980) who states that in the case of chronic pain TT should be used in conjunction with counselling. With conditions such as chronic pain it may take a number of sessions before the energy flow is rebalanced and maintained in harmony (Owens & Ehrenreich, 1991a).

Owens and Ehrenreich (1991b) suggest that because TT does not require any physical contact with the skin there are times when it is particularly useful. For example in patients who are unable to tolerate physical contact, such as those with burns or those who do not liked to be touched, TT provides an acceptable non-pharmacological intervention which may make a contribution to pain relief.

8.4 Transcutaneous electrical nerve stimulation (TENS)

Nerves act by conducting electrical impulses and conversely we can apply electrical impulses to a nerve to alter the way in which it fires. In principle, we should like to stimulate A-beta nerve fibres and thus block any impulses coming from the nociceptive A-delta and C-fibres (see Chapter 2). Although we cannot pick out the precise fibres to stimulate, the technique of using electrical impulses to block nociceptive transmission does work, as does the use of massage, rubbing or ice and heat to produce the same effect.

When the techniques of stimulating nerves with electricity first started, electrodes had to be implanted in physical contact with the nerve. For some kinds of severe intractable pain electrode implantation is still used. However, in 1967 Norman Shealy, a neurosurgeon who had been implanting electrodes, discovered that devices that transmitted electricity transcutaneously were just as effective. This observation increased enormously the potential of using electrical impulses to control pain and the modern day technique of transcutaneous electrical nerve stimulation or TENS was born.

Despite thirty years of successful use, TENS is still rather a haphazard technique and relies on finding the correct placement of electrodes and correct pattern of electrical stimulation by trial and error rather than any well defined guidelines for use. A TENS unit consists of a power source, usually a battery and electrodes, to be placed over or near the site of the pain. The battery can deliver electrical impulses which will be continuous or pulsed; and the pulse waveform, frequency, pattern, width and duration must all be chosen to suit the individual. The selection of these parameters is empirical, the unit must be tried at a variety of different settings and seems to depend as much on the experience of the person administering the TENS as anything else.

As a rough guide most units work with maximum currents of around 60 milliamperes, delivered for about 250 microseconds; most outputs are biphasic. Studies have shown that endorphins are only released at pulses of 8 Hz or less. Wider pulses spread the current over greater distances; the ranges in most TENS units are from 50 to 400 milliseconds. Thus closely placed electrodes can have small pulse widths, and the further apart the electrodes are, the wider the pulse width should be.

Electrode placement is also very important in obtaining optimal effects. In general the electrodes are placed 'between the pain and the brain' along nerve roots, dermatomes of the respective nerve levels, following the pathway of referred pain or on trigger points. Sometimes an electrode over a trigger point will increase the pain (since the trigger point is the area where pressure will simulate the pain – see Chapter 3). If this occurs, treating across the area, about 3-4 cm either side with microstimulation of 0.5 Hz will almost always alleviate it.

Electrodes are usually self-adhesive and in this age of concern over transmission of infection, usually semi-disposable or at least separate sets are kept for individual patients.

Because of the 'trial and error' nature of the stimulating parameters, it often takes some time to obtain success with TENS. But for some patients the perseverance may be worthwhile; and once the correct parameters are achieved, it is a handy portable pain relief system that can be self-administered by the patient. There are few contra-indications to TENS, although it is essential that electrodes are not placed on the head or neck, especially over the carotid sinus where stimulation could cause a vago-vagal syncope (fainting due to lack of blood to the brain). TENS should not be used in people with cardiac pacemakers.

A more detailed discussion of the electrical parameters and settings for TENS equipment is given in Johnson *et al.* (1991); McDevitt (1995) gives photographically illustrated instructions on the use of TENS equipment.

8.5 Acupuncture and acupressure

Acupuncture

Acupuncture is an ancient form of medicine practised by the Chinese for hundreds of years. The Chinese believe that meridians exist which connect internal parts of the body to accessible cutaneous sites. Vital energy circulates in these meridians. Stimulation of these sites can reduce pain, relieve symptoms or cure diseases which are present along these meridians. Maps of these meridians have been in existence for hundreds of years. As Western science has not been able to find any physiological basis for these maps, the technique has met with some scepticism in the West. However, there is a remarkably high correlation between trigger point sites and acupuncture points; 70% of trigger points correspond to acupuncture sites (Melzack *et al.*, 1977).

Acupuncture has also been proposed to stimulate release of endorphins (Belgrade, 1994; Pomeranz 1994), to modulate pain producing neurotransmitters (Belgrade, 1994; Pomeranz, 1994; Vincent & Lewith, 1994) or to produce stress-induced analgesia (Clark, 1994). Even if we cannot prove how it works, for those who believe in acupuncture it can be very useful. Belief in the technique may be important in its effectiveness.

The location of the correct acupuncture point for a particular pain and administration of acupuncture can usually only be carried out by someone trained in the technique. Needles are then inserted which are twisted, heated or stimulated electrically to stimulate the acupuncture point.

Acupressure

The non-invasive form of acupuncture is acupressure where pressure is applied to the relevant acupuncture point without puncturing the skin. This has the advantage that once an effective site has been identified acupressure can be used by nurses, other health care professionals or carers. Since meridians flow in a particular direction, acupressure is usually applied as massage in the direction of flow. A comprehensive guide to the uses of acupressure is to be found in Kenyon (1988).

Summary of Chapter 8

- Cognitive-behavioural strategies include a range of different interventions which are aimed at changing the patient's perception of pain, altering dysfunctional pain behaviours and fostering a sense of control over pain.
- Distraction involves patients focusing their attention on to a stimulus other than their pain, thereby pushing the pain to the periphery of their awareness.
- Focusing is a cognitive coping technique where patients make a deliberate effort to focus on their pain and imagine different ways of controlling that pain.
- Reframing helps patients to identify and correct distorted perception, misinterpretations, unrealistic expectations, and irrational beliefs about pain.
- Hypnosis is a very sophisticated and complex way of bringing about a relaxation response and is normally administered by a trained therapist.
- Guided imagery is a cognitive technique which involves using one's mind to create or experience a mental image which in turn either distracts attention away from the pain experience or focuses attention directly on to the pain.
- Biofeedback is a technique where the person uses some form of auditory or visual signal to increase awareness of how he or she is responding in a stressful situation. The person is thought to relax in response to that signal.
- Cutaneous stimulation includes a range of non-invasive methods which are thought to either increase transmission of non-noxious inputs into the spinal cord or to modulate the transmission of noxious inputs, both of which result in varying degrees of pain control.
- Massage involves the stimulation of the skin and underlying tissues with varying degrees of hand pressure.
- Aromatherapy involves the use of aromatic essential oils to ameliorate pain.
- Superficial application of heat and cold are thought to ameliorate pain by relaxing muscle spasm, reducing joint stiffness and decreasing muscle tone. Efficacy may be improved by using them alternately.
- Therapeutic touch is thought to correct imbalances in an individual's energy field which have been disrupted by ill-health. There is limited scientific evidence to support TT; but if patients find it helpful, it can be a useful technique.
- Transcutaneous nerve stimulation uses electrical impulses to block nociceptive transmission.
- Acupuncture is an ancient form of Chinese medicine which involves stimulation of cutaneous and subcutaneous sites (which are thought to represent deeper tissues) with needles to bring about pain relief.
- Acupressure is the non-invasive form of acupuncture where pressure is applied to the acupuncture point rather than puncturing the skin.

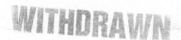

Glossary

Acetyl choline The neurotransmitter at some sympathetic and all para-sympathetic synapses. Such synapses are termed cholinergic.

Action potential A short-lasting change in electrical activity that propagates messages along a nerve. An action potential is caused by movement of charged ions across a nerve membrane which results in a change in the electrical potential of that membrane

Addiction (to a drug) Physical and/or psychological dependence on a drug characterised by a craving for the drug. People can be addicted to things other than drugs – e.g. food, behaviours.

Adjuvant Assisting or aiding.

Afferent Afferent nerves transmit information from the periphery to the central nervous system.

Agonist Ligand which stimulates normal activity at a receptor.

Allodynia Increased sensitivity to pain such that stimuli which are normally innocuous produce pain.

Analgesia Absence of pain on noxious stimulation or suppression of pain.

Analgesic Substance or technique that reduces pain.

Analogue Structurally related or similar.

Antagonist Ligand which prevents normal activity at a receptor.

Anterior commissure Area of spinal cord (at the front) that connects the right and left sides.

Antidromic (antidromically) Nerve conduction in the opposite direction to normal.

Anti-tussive A drug that prevents coughing.

Apnoea (apnea) Cessation of breathing.

Atrophy Wasting away.

Autonomic Division of the nervous system that controls functions over which we do not usually have conscious control – e.g. digestion, heart beat.

Axon Fine projection of nerve cells which conduct impulses away from the cell body.

Brainstem The most posterior region of the brain, connecting cerebral hemispheres to the spinal cord. Consists of pons, medulla and midbrain.

Breakthrough pain Pain caused by movement, pressure, flatulence, treatment intervention or low plasma level of analgesics.

Causalgia Sympathetically maintained pain of burning nature.

Central pain   Pain associated with a lesion of the CNS.

Co-analgesics   Drugs used in conjunction with analgesics to relieve pain.

Congener   A person or thing of the same kind or nature. Congeners of morphine will be isolated along with morphine during extraction procedures.

Cordotomy   Severing of the spinal cord.

Cryocoagulation   Destruction of tissue by extreme cold.

CSF   Cerebro-spinal fluid.

Dynorphin   Endogenous opiate involved in analgesia.

Dysaesthesia   Unpleasant, abnormal sensation produced by normal stimuli.

Dysphoria   Disquiet, feelings of unreality.

Efferent   Relaying information from the CNS to the periphery.

Ephapse nerves   Abnormal electrical contacts between afferent nociceptive and efferent sympathetic nerves.

Euphoria   Feeling of well being, extreme happiness.

Equianalgesic   Producing the same degree of analgesia.

Fibrosis   Formation of thickened, scar like, tissue.

First-pass metabolism   Metabolism of a drug that occurs during its first pass through the liver. Agents absorbed from the gut pass through the liver before entering the systemic circulation and are therefore subject to first-pass metabolism.

Focal   Localised to a specific area.

Hyperalgesia   Increased sensitivity to pain or noxious stimulation.

Hyperasthesia   Increased sensitivity to stimulation, excluding the special senses.

Hyperpathia   A painful syndrome, characterised by prolonged response to a stimulus after it has been removed.

Hyperpolarised   Of cells, where the membrane potential has been raised. In a nerve cell this will result in action potentials being induced more easily.

Hypopolarised   Lowered membrane potential – hence less easily activated nerve cell.

Indication   Condition or reason for which the use of a drug has been approved.

Incident pain   Pain produced by an incident such as moving.

Lancinating   Sharp, cutting, shooting – used to describe pain.

Limbic system   Basal system of the brain associated with emotion and behaviour.

Mast cells   Cell involved in inflammatory response. Releases a variety of inflammatory mediators, notably histamine.

Neuroma (pl. neuromata)   Tangle of nerve fibres formed when a severed nerve is unsuccessful in reinnervating the area of tissue it previously supplied.

Neuralgia   Pain in the distribution of a nerve or nerves.

Neuritis   Inflammation of a nerve or nerves.

Neuropathy   A disturbance of function or pathological change in a nerve. (One nerve – mononeuropathy; several nerves – mono-neuropathy multiplex; bilateral and symmetrical – polyneuoropathy).

Nociceptor   A receptor sensitive to noxious stimuli.

Noxious   Damaging to tissue.

Percutaneous   Through the skin.

Peritoneum   Membrane lining the abdominal cavity.

Pain   An unpleasant sensory and emotional experience associated with actual or potential tissue damage, or described in terms of such damage (IASP definition).

Postsynaptic   Area after the synaptic cleft. The region on to which the information is being passed.

Postsynaptic neurone   Neurone receiving information across the synapse.

Presynaptic   Area before the synapse, that is, on the side of the synapse receiving the message.

Presynaptic neurone   Neurone passing on information across the synapse.

Prophylactic   Preventative, in anticipation of.

Proprioception   The sensation or identification of where the body is in space.

Pruritus   Itching.

Psychogenic   Arising in the mind.

Psychomimetic   Mimicking psychoses.

Psychotropic   Having an effect on the mind.

Plexus   A network (usually of nerves).

Radicular   Pertaining to a nerve root.

Radiculopathy   Disease of nerve root.

Refractory   Not responsive to treatment.

Remission   Halting or containing disease process. Reduction of symptoms.

Rescue medication   Medication given to relieve symptoms when they are not controlled by usual medication.

Spino-thalamic tract   Ascending pathway which transmits nociceptive information coming from the periphery via the spinal cord to the thalamus in the brain.

Substantia gelatinosa   The central structure of the spinal cord. H-shaped, it has a jelly-like appearance in fresh tissue.

Synapse   Small gap between a nerve ending and the next cell. Neurotransmitters are the means whereby information is passed across this gap.

Syringomelia   A disease of the spinal cord in which longitudinal cavities form in the cervical region, damaging motor nerve cells and fibres that transmit sensations of pain and temperature, resulting in wasting and lack of sensation in one arm and hand.

Tenesmus   Unproductive straining to defecate.

TENS   Transcutaneous Electrical Nerve Stimulation.

Thalamus   Part of brain between hypothalamus and limbic system. Involved in relay of sensory information to the cortex. Involved in pain perception and arousal.

References

Abu-Saad, H.H., Pool, H. & Tulkens, B. (1994) Further validity testing of the Abu-Saad Paediatric Pain Assessment Tool. *Journal of Advanced Nursing*, **19**, 1063–1071.

Agency for Health Care Policy and Research (1992) *Acute Pain Management: Operative or Medical Procedures and Trauma.* AHCPR Publication no. 92–0032. U.S. Department of Health and Human Services, Rockville, MD.

Ahles, T.A., Ruckdeschel, J.C. & Blanchard, B. (1984) Cancer-related pain – 1. Prevalence in outpatient setting as a function of stage of disease and type of cancer. *Journal of Psychosomatic Research*, **28**, 115–119.

Akil, M. & Amos, R.S. (1995) ABC of rheumatology: rheumatoid arthritis – I: Clinical features and diagnosis. *British Medical Journal*, **310**, 587–590.

Al Absi, M. & Rokke, P.D. (1991) Can anxiety help us tolerate pain? *Pain*, **46**, 43–51.

Alderdice, F. & Marchant, S. (1997) Water in labour. In: *Understanding Pain and Its Relief in Labour* (ed. S. Moore), pp. 113–128. Churchill Livingstone, Edinburgh.

Alleyne, J. & Thomas, V.J. (1994) The management of sickle cell crisis pain as experienced by patients and carers. *Journal of Advanced Nursing*, **19**, 725–732.

Angus, J.E. & Faux, S. (1989) The effects of music on adult post-operative patients' pain during a nursing procedure. In: *Management of Pain, Fatigue and Nausea* (eds S.G. Funk, E.M. Tornquist, M.T. Champagne, L.A. Copp & R.A. Wise), pp. 166–172. Springer Publishing Company, New York.

Anon (1979) Pain Terms: a list with definitions and notes on usage. Recommended by the IASP subcommittee on taxonomy. *Pain*, **6**, 249–252.

Arathuzik, M.D. (1991) The appraisal of pain and coping in cancer patients. *Western Journal of Nursing Research*, **13**, 714–731.

Arathuzik, M.D. (1994) Effects of cognitive-behavioral strategies on pain in cancer patients. *Cancer Nursing*, **17** (3), 207–214.

Arner, S. & Meyerson, B.A. (1988) Lack of analgesic effect of opioids on neuropathic and ideopathic forms of pain. *Pain*, **37**, 335–346.

Aronson, J.K. (1991) Routes of drug administration: 1. Rectal. *Prescribers Journal*, **31** (3), 93–97.

Aronson, J.K. (1995) Routes of drug administration: 5. Intramuscular injection. *Prescribers Journal*, **35** (1), 32–36.

Atkins, R.M. & Duthie, R.B. (1987) Algodystrophy (reflex sympathetic dystrophy or Sudeck's atrophy). In: *Oxford Textbook of Medicine* (eds D.J. Weatherall, J.G.G. Ledingham, D.A.Warrel), pp. 16.89–16.91, Second Edition. Oxford Medical Publications, OUP, Oxford.

Austin, C., Cody, C.P., Eyers, P.J., Hefferin, E.A. & Krasnow, R.W. (1986)

Hospice home care pain management: four critical variables. *Cancer Nursing*, 9 (2), 58–65.

Averill, P.M., Novy, D.M., Nelson, D.V. & Berry, L.A. (1996) Correlates of depression in chronic pain patients: a comprehensive examination. *Pain*, 65, 93–100.

Baines, M. & Sykes, N. (1993) Gastrointestinal symptoms. In: *Management of Terminal Malignant Disease*, 3rd edn (eds C. Saunders & N. Sykes), pp. 63–75. Edward Arnold, London.

Ballantyne, J.C., Loach, A.B. & Carr, D.B. (1988) Itching after epidural and spinal opiates. *Pain*, 33, 149–160.

Bamfield, T. (1997) Management of labour pain by midwives: a historical perspective. In: *Understanding Pain and Its Relief in Labour* (ed. S. Moore), pp. 63–76, Churchill Livingstone, Edinburgh.

Barkwell, D.P. (1991) Ascribed meaning: a critical factor in coping and pain attenuation in patients with cancer-related pain. *Journal of Palliative Care*, 7, 5–14.

Bates, M.S., Edwards, W.T. & Anderson, K.O. (1993) Ethnocultural influences on variation in chronic pain perception. *Pain*, 52, 101–112.

Baumann, A. & Deber, R. (1989) *Decision Making and Problem Solving in Nursing: An Overview of the Relevant Literature*, Literature Review Monograph 3. University of Toronto, Toronto.

Beecher, H.K. (1956) Relationship of significance of wound to pain experienced. *Journal of the American Medical Association*, 161, 1609–1613.

Bélanger, E., Melzack, R. & Lauzon, P. (1989) Pain of first-trimester abortion: a study of psychosocial and medical predictors. *Pain*, 36, 339–350.

Belgrade, M. (1994) Two decades after ping-pong diplomacy: is there a role for acupuncture in American pain medicine? *APS J*, 3, 73–83.

Bendelow, G.A. & Williams, S.J. (1995) Transcending the dualism: towards a sociology of pain. *Sociology of Health and Illness*, 17 (2), 139–165.

Benson, H. & Friedman, R. (1996) Harnessing the power of the placebo effect and renaming it 'remembered wellness'. *Annual Review of Medicine*, 47, 193–199.

Bergbom Engberg, A., Grondahl, G. & Thibom, K. (1995) Patients' experiences of herpes zoster and postherpetic neuralgia. *Journal of Advanced Nursing*, 3, 427–433.

Bogduk, N. (1989) Understanding pain pathways. *Current Therapeutics*, 1, 25–40.

Boguslawski, M. (1980) Therapeutic touch: a facilitator of pain relief. *Topics in Clinical Nursing*, 2 (1), 27–37.

Bond, M.R. (1980) The suffering of severe intractable pain. In: *Pain and Society* (eds H.A. Kosterlitz, L.Y. Terenius), pp. 53–62. Verlag Chemie, Weinheim.

Bond, S. & Pearson, I.B. (1969) Psychological aspects of pain in women with advanced cancer of the cervix. *Journal of Psychosomatic Research*, 13, 13–19.

Bonica, J.J. (1994) Labour pain. In: *Textbook of Pain* (eds P.D. Wall & R. Melzack), pp. 615–642. Churchill Livingstone, Edinburgh.

Boore, J. (1978) *Prescription for Recovery*. Royal College of Nursing, London.

Borenstein, D.G. & Wiesel, S.W. (1989) *Low Back Pain*. W.B. Saunders Company, Philadelphia.

Bourbonnais, F. (1981) Pain assessment: development of a tool for the nurse and the patient. *Journal of Advanced Nursing*, 6, 227–282.

Bozzette, M. (1993). Observation of pain behaviour in the NICU: An exploratory study. *Journal of Perinatal and Neonatal Nursing*, 7, 76–87.

Brandt, J. (1995) The use of access devices in cancer pain control, *Seminars in Oncology Nursing*, 11 (3), 203–212.

Brattberg, G., Thorslund, M. & Wikman, A. (1989) The prevalance of pain in a general population: the results of a postal survey in a county of Sweden. *Pain*, 37, 215–222.

Breneis, C., Michaud, M., Bruera, E. & MacDonald, R.N. (1987) Local toxicity during the subcutaneous infusion of narcotics (SCIN). *Cancer Nursing*, 10 (4), 172–176.

Breivik, H. & Rennemo, F. (1982) Clinical evaluation of a combined treatment with methadone and pyschotropic drugs in cancer patients. *Acta Aanethetica Scandinavica*, Suppl 74, 135–140.

Broome, M.E., Lillis, P.P., McGahee, T.W. & Bates, T. (1992) The use of distraction and imagery with children during painful procedures. *Oncology Nursing Forum*, 19, 499–502.

Brownridge, P. (1995) The nature and consequences of childbirth pain. *European Journal of Obstetrics, Gynaecology and Reproductive Biology*, 59 (Suppl), S9–15.

Bruera, E., Kuehn, N., Miller, M.J., Selmser, P. & Macmillan, K. (1991) The Edmonton Symptom Assessment System (ESAS): a simple method for the assessment of palliative care patients. *Journal of Palliative Care*, 7, 6–9.

Bruera, E. & Watanabe, S. (1994) New developments in the assessment of pain in cancer patients. *Supportive Care in Cancer*, 2, 312–318.

Buckley, M.M. & Benfield, P. (1993) Eutectic lidocaine/prilocaine cream. A review of the topical anaesthetic/analgesic efficacy of a eutectic mixture of local anaesthetics (EMLA). *Drugs*, 46, 126–151.

Bush, F.M., Harkins, S.W., Harrington, W.G. & Price, D.D. (1993) Analysis of gender effects on pain perception and symptom presentation in temporomandibular pain. *Pain*, 53, 73–80.

Butler, R.H. (1975) *Why Survive? Being Old in America*. Harper & Row, New York.

Canty, S.L. (1994) Constipation as a side effect of opioids. *Oncology Nursing Forum*, 21, 739–745.

Camp, L.D. (1988) A comparison of nurses' recorded assessments of pain with perceptions as described by cancer patients. *Cancer Nursing*, 11, 237–243.

Camp-Sorrell, D. & O'Sullivan, P. (1991) Effects of continuing education: pain assessment and documentation. *Cancer Nursing*, 14, 49–54.

Carlen, P.L., Wall, P.D., Nadvorna, H. & Steinbach, T. (1978) Phantom limbs and related phenomena in recent traumatic amputation. *Neurology* (Minneap.), 28, 211–217.

Carr, E. (1990) Postoperative pain: patient's expectations and experiences. *Journal of Advanced Nursing*, 15, 89–100.

Cassel, E.J. (1982) The nature of suffering and the goals of medicine. *New England Journal of Medicine*, 306, 639–645.

Cervero, F. (1991) Mechanism of acute visceral pain. *British Medical Bulletin*, 47, 549–560.

Chapman, C.R., Casey, K.L., Dubner, R., Foley, K.M., Gracely, R.H. & Reading, A.E. (1985) Pain measurement: an overview. *Pain*, 22, 1–31.

Cherny, N.I. & Portenoy, R.K. (1994) Cancer pain: principles of assessment and syndromes. In: *Textbook of pain* (eds P.D. Wall & R. Melzack), 3rd edn, pp. 787–824. Churchill Livingstone, Edinburgh.

Choiniere, M., Melzack, R., Girard, N., Rondeau, J. & Paquin, M.-J. (1990) Comparisons between patients' and nurses' assessment of pain and medication efficacy in severe burn injuries. *Pain*, **40**, 143–152.

Cianciolo Livingston, J. (1985) The use of music and exercise to reduce the pain of pregnancy and childbirth. In: *Recent Advances in Nursing: Perspectives on Pain* (ed. L.A. Copp), pp. 92–112. Churchill Livingstone, Edinburgh.

Clark, W.C. (1994) Acupuncture and other 'alternative medicine' therapies. *APS J*, **3**, 84–88.

Closs, S. (1994) Pain in elderly patients: a neglected phenomenon? *Journal of Advanced Nursing*, **19**, 1072–1081.

Closs, S. (1996) Pain and elderly patients: a survey of nurses' knowledge and experiences. *Journal of Advanced Nursing*, **23**, 237–242.

Coderre, T.J., Melzack, R. (1992) The contribution of excitatory amino acids to central sensitization and persistent nociception after formalin-induced tissue injury. *Journal of Neuroscience*, **12**, 3665–70.

Coe, C. (1997) Advances in nursing patients with intractable pain. *Contemporary Nurse*, **6**, 32–39.

Cogan, R. (1978) Practice time in prepared childbirth. *Journal of Obstetric and Gynaecological Nursing*, **23**, 17–21.

Cogan, R. & Spinnato, J.A. (1986) Pain and discomfort thresholds in late pregnancy. *Pain*, **27**, 63–68.

Cohen, F. (1980) Postsurgical pain relief: patients' status and nurses' medication choices. *Pain*, **9**, 265–274.

Commission of the European Communities (1990) Proposal for a Council Directive concerning the legal status for the supply of medicinal products for human use. COM (89) 607 final. *Official Journal of the European Communities*, Brussels.

Cooper, K. & Bennett, W. (1987) Nephrotoxicity of common drugs used in clinical practice. *Archives of Intern Medicine*, **147**, 1231–1218.

Copp, L.A. (1974) The spectrum of suffering. *American Journal of Nursing*, **3**, 491–495.

Copp, L.A. (1990) An AJN classic: The spectrum of suffering. *American Journal of Nursing*, **8**, 35–39.

Couvreur, C. (1990) *Palliative Care in Europe*. European Commission's Europe Against Cancer Programme, Brussels.

Coyle, N., Adelhardt, J. & Foley, K.M. (1990) Character of terminal illness in the advanced cancer patient: pain and other symptoms in the last four weeks of life. *Journal of Pain and Symptom Management*, **5**, 83–89.

Coyle, N., Cherny, N. & Portenoy, R.K. (1995) Pharmacologic management of cancer pain. In: *Cancer Pain Management*, 2nd edn (eds D.B. McGuire, C. Henke Yarbro & B.R. Ferrell), pp. 89–130. Jones and Bartlett Publishers, Boston.

Cox, T. (1978) *Stress*. Macmillan, London.

Crook, J., Rideout, E. & Browne, G. (1984) The prevalence of pain complaints in a general population. *Pain*, **18**, 299–314.

Crosby, G., Marota, J.J., Goto T. & Uhl, G.R. (1994) Subarachnoid morphine reduces stimulation-induced but not basal expression of proenkephalin in rat spinal cord. *Anesthesiology*, **81**, 1270–6.

Cruise, C.E., Broderick, J., Porter, L., Kaell, A. & Stone, A.A. (1996) Reactive effects of diary self-assessment in chronic pain patients. *Pain*, **67**, 253–258.

Dale, A. & Cornwell, S. (1994) The role of lavender oil in relieving perineal discomfort following childbirth. *Journal of Advanced Nursing*, **19** (1), 89–96.

Dalton, J.A. (1989) Nurses' perception of their pain assessment skills, pain management practices, and attitudes towards pain. *Oncology Nursing Forum*, **16** (2), 225–231.

Daut, R.L. & Cleelend, C.S. (1982) The prevalence and severity of pain in cancer. *Cancer*, **50**, 197–210.

Daut, R.L., Cleeland, C.S. & Flanery, R.C. (1983) The development of the Wisconsin Brief Pain Questionnaire to assess pain in cancer and other diseases. *Pain*, **17**, 197–210.

Davies, I., Gangar, K.F., Drummond, M., Saunders, D. & Beard, R.W. (1992) The economic burden of intractable gynaecological pain. *Journal of Obstetrics and Gynaecology*, Suppl 2, 54–6.

Davies, R. (1997) Transcutaneous Electrical Nerve Stimulation. In: *Understanding Pain and Its Relief in Labour* (ed. S. Moore), pp. 129–148, Churchill Livingstone, Edinburgh.

Davies, S. & Riches, L. (1995) Healing touch? *Nursing Times*, **91** (25), 42–43.

Davis, B.D. (1984) Pre-operative Information Giving and Patients' Post-operative Outcomes: an Implementation Study. Unpublished Report. Nursing Research Unit, University of Edinburgh.

Davis, B.D., Billings, J. & Ryland, R.K. (1994) Evaluation of nursing process documentation. *Journal of Advanced Nursing*, **19**, 960–968.

Davis, P.S. (1988) Changing nursing practice for more effective control of post-operative pain through a staff initiated educational programme. *Nurse Education Today*, **8**, 325–331.

Davitz, L.L.& Davitz, J.R. (1985) Culture and nurses' inferences of suffering. In: *Recent Advances in Nursing: Perspectives on Pain* (ed. L.A. Copp), pp. 17–28. Churchill Livingstone, Edinburgh.

Dean, F.M. (1989) The chemical classification of azapropazone. In: *Azaprone – 20 years of clinical use* (ed. K.D. Rainsford), pp. 9–19. Kluwer, Lancaster, UK.

De Conno, F. & Foley, K. (1995) *Cancer Pain Relief: A Practical Manual*. Kluwer Academic Publishers, Dordrecht.

de la Cuesta, C. (1983) The nursing process: from development to implementation. *Journal of Advanced Nursing*, **8**, 365–371.

de Stoutz, N.D., Bruera, E. & Suarez-Almazor, M. (1995) Opioid rotation for toxicity reduction in terminal cancer patients. *Journal of Pain and Symptom Management*, **10**, 378–384.

Deschamps, M., Band, P.R. & Coldman, A.J. (1988) Assessment of adult cancer pain: shortcomings of current methods. *Pain*, **32**, 133–139.

Diekmann, J.M. & Wassem, R.A. (1991) A survey of nursing students' knowledge of cancer pain control. *Cancer Nursing*, **14**, 314–320.

Dieppe, P. (1987) Osteoarthritis and related disorders. In: *Oxford Textbook of Medicine* (eds D.J. Wetherall, J.G.G. Ledingham & D.A. Warrell), 2nd Edition. Oxford Medical Publications, Oxford.

Donovan, M., Dillon, P. & McGuire, L. (1987) Incidence and characteristics of pain in a sample of medical-surgical patients. *Pain*, 30, 69–78.

Donovan, M. (1989) Relieving pain: the current basis for practice. In: *Management of Pain, Fatigue and Nausea* (eds S. G. Funk, E.M. Tornquist, M.T. Champagne, L.A. Copp & R.A. Wise), pp. 25–29. Springer Publishing Company, New York.

Draisci, G. & Iadarola, M.J. (1989) Temporal analysis of increases in c-*fos*, preprodynorphin and preproenkephalin mRNAs in rat spinal cord. *Molecular Brain Research*, 6, 31–37.

Duchene, P. (1989) The effectiveness of biofeedback in relieving childbirth pain. In: *Management of Pain, Fatigue and Nausea* (eds S. G. Funk, E.M. Tornquist, M.T. Champagne, L.A. Copp & R.A. Wise), pp. 145–150. Springer Publishing Company, New York.

Dudley, S.R. & Holm, K. (1984) Assessment of the pain experience in relation to selected nurse characteristics. *Pain*, 18, 179–186.

Dufault, M.A., Bielecki, C., Collins, E. & Willey, C. (1995) Changing nurses' pain assessment practice: a collaborative research utilization approach. *Journal of Advanced Nursing*, 21, 634–645.

Duggan, A.W. (1985) Pharamacology of descending control systems. *Phil Trans Roy Soc Lond (B)*, 308, 375–391.

Eland, J.M. (1978) Living with pain. *Nursing Outlook*, July, 430–431.

Eland, J.M. (1985) The role of the nurse in children's pain. In: *Recent Advances in Nursing: Perspectives on Pain* (ed. L.A. Copp), pp. 29–45. Churchill Livingstone, Edinburgh.

Ellis, R.M. (1995) Back pain. *British Medical Journal*, 310, 1220.

Ernst, E. & Fialka, V. (1994) Ice freezes pain? A review of the clinical effectiveness of analgesic cold therapy. *Journal of Pain and Symptom Management*, 9 (1), 56–59.

European Commission's Europe Against Cancer Programme (1993) Report of a Subcommittee on Palliative Cancer Care, DOC.DG.V.E. 1/6002/93, Brussels.

Evely, L. (1967) *Suffering*. Herder and Herder, New York.

Fagerhaugh, S.Y. & Strauss, A. (1977) *Politics of Pain Management: Staff-Patient Interaction*. Addison-Wesley, California.

Feine, J.S., Bushnell, M.C., Miron, D. & Duncan, G.H. (1991) Sex differences in the perception of noxious heat stimuli. *Pain*, 44, 255–262.

Ferrell, B.A., Ferrell, B.R. & Osterweil, D. (1990) Pain in the nursing home. *Journal of American Geriatric Society*, 39, 409–414.

Ferrell, B.A., Zichi Cohen, M., Rhiner, M. & Rozek, A. (1991) Pain as a metaphor for illness. Part 11: family caregivers' management of pain. *Oncology Nursing Forum*, 18 (8), 1315–1321.

Ferrell, B.A. & Dean, G. (1995) The meaning of cancer pain. *Seminars in Oncology Nursing*, 11 (1), 17–22.

Ferrell, B.R., Grant, M., Chan, J., Ahn, C. & Ferrell, B.A. (1995) The impact of cancer pain education on family caregivers of elderly patients. *Oncology Nursing Forum*, 22 (8), 1211–1218.

Ferrel, B., Wisdom, C., Wenzl, C. & Brown, J. (1989). Effects of controlled release morphine on quality of life for cancer patients. *Oncology Nursing Forum*, 16, 521–525.

Ferrel-Torry, A. & Glick, O. (1993) The use of therapeutic massage as a nursing intervention to modify anxiety and the perception of cancer pain. *Cancer Nursing*, 16 (2), 93–101.

Ferriera, S.H., Lorenzetti, B.B., Bristow, A.F., & Poole, S. (1988) Interleukin -1ß as a potent hyperalgesic agent antagonised by a tripeptide analogue. *Nature*, 334, 698–700.

Fields, H.L.(1987). *Pain*. McGraw-Hill, New York.

Findlay, J.W.A., Jones, E.C., Butz, R.F. & Welch, R.M. (1978) Plasma codeine and morphine concentrations after therapeutic doses of codeine-containing analgesics. *Clin. Pharm. Therapy*, 24, 60–68.

Fishman, B. & Loscalzo, M. (1987) Cognitive-behavioral interventions in management of cancer pain: principles and applications. *Medical Clinics of North America*, 71 (2), 271–287.

Foley, K.M. (1979) The management of pain of malignant origin. In: *Current Neurology* Vol 2 (eds Tyler, H.R. & Dawson, D.M.), pp. 279–302. Houghton Mifflin, Boston, MA.

Foley, K.M. (1993) Pain assessment and cancer pain syndromes. In: *Oxford Textbook of Palliative Medicine* (eds D. Doyle, G.W.C. Hanks & N. MacDonald), Chapter 4.2.2. pp. 148–165. Oxford Medical Publications, Oxford.

Foley, K. & Inturrisi, C. (1992) *Opioid Therapy: General Principles, Advances, Controversies, Alternative Routes and Methods of Administration.* Syllabus of the Postgraduate Course, Memorial Sloan-Kettering Cancer Center, 2–4 April, New York.

Fordham, M. & Dunn, V. (1994) *Alongside the Person in Pain.* Balliere Tindall, London.

Foster, R.W. & Cox, B. (1983) *Basic Pharmacology.* Butterworths, London.

Fothergill-Bourbonnais, F. & Wilson-Barnett, J. (1992) A comparative study of intensive therapy unit and hospice nurses' knowledge on pain management. *Journal of Advanced Nursing*, 17, 362–372.

Fox, L. (1982) Pain management in the terminally ill cancer patient: an investigation of nurses' attitudes, knowledge and clinical practice. *Military Medicine*, 147 (6), 455–459.

Francke, A.L. & Theeuwen, I. (1994) Inhibition in expressing pain: a qualitative study among Dutch surgical breast cancer patients. *Cancer Nursing*, 17 (3), 193–199.

Friedrichs, J.B., Young, S., Gallagher, D., Keller, C. & Kimura, R.E. (1995) Where does it hurt? An interdisciplinary approach to improving the quality of pain assessment and management in the neonatal intensive care unit. *Nursing Clinics of North America*, 30 (1), 143–157.

Garro, L. (1990) Culture, pain and cancer. *Journal of Palliative Care*, 6 (3), 34–44.

Gaskin, M.E., Greene, A.F., Robinson, M.E. & Geisser, M.E. (1992) Negative affect and the experience of chronic pain. *Journal of Psychosomatic Research*, 36 (8), 707–713.

Gintzler, A.R. (1980) Endorphin-mediated increases in pain threshold during pregnancy. *Science*, 210, 193–195.

Gleeson, B. (1991) Loosening the grip of anginal pain. *Nursing*, 21 (1), 33–40.

Goodwin, J.S. & Regan, M. (1982) Cognitive dysfunction associated with naproxen and ibuprofen in the elderly. *Arthritis and Rheumatism*, 25, 1013–1015.

Gordon, M. (1987) *Nursing Diagnosis: Process and Application.* McGraw-Hill, New York.

Gould, T.H., Crosby, D.L., Harmer, M., Lloyd, S.M., Lunn, J.N., Rees, G.A.D., Roberts, D.E. & Webster, J.A. (1992) Policy for controlling pain after surgery: effect of sequential changes in management. *British Journal of Medicine*, 305, 1187–1193.

Gourlay, G.K., Cherry, D.A. & Cousins, M.J. (1985) Cephalad migration of morphine in CSF following lumbar epidural administration in patients with cancer pain. *Pain*, 23, 317–326.

Grahn, G. & Johnson, J. (1990) Learning to cope and living with cancer. Learning needs assessment in cancer patient education. *Scandanavian Journal of Caring Science*, 4 (4).

Gray, M.A. (1991) Morphine: an old drug reviewed and reexamined. *Orthopaedic Nursing*, 10, 63–67.

Greenwald, H.P. (1991) Interethnic differences in pain perception. *Pain*, 44, 157–163.

Grigg, P., Schaible, H-G. & Schmid, R.F. (1986). Mechanical sensitivity of group II and IV afferents from the posterior articular nerve in normal and inflammed cat knee. *Journal of Neurophysiology*, 55, 635–643.

Grossman, S.A., Sheidler, V.R., Swedeen, K., Mucenski, J. & Piantasosi, S. (1991) Correlation of patient and caregiver ratings of cancer pain. *Journal of Pain and Symptom Management*, 6, 53–57.

Haldeman, S. (1994) Manipulation and massage for the relief of back pain. In: *Textbook of Pain* (eds P.D. Wall & R. Melzack), 3rd edition, pp. 1251–1262. Churchill Livingstone, Edinburgh.

Hamers, J.P.H., Abu-Saad, H.H., van den Hout, M.A. *et al.* (1996) The influence of children's vocal expressions, age, medical diagnosis and information obtained from parents on nurses' pain assessments and decisions regarding interventions. *Pain*, 65, 53–61.

Hammack, J.E. & Loprinzi, C.L. (1994) Use of orally administered opioids for cancer-related pain. *Mayo Clinics Proceedings*, 69, 384–390.

Hanks, G.W., Hoskin, P.J., Aherne, G.W., Turner, P. & Poulain, P. (1987) Explanation for potency of repeated oral doses of morphine? *Lancet*, ii, 723–725.

Hanks, G.W., Portenoy, R.K., MacDonald, N. & O'Neill, W.M. (1993) Difficult pain problems. In *Oxford Textbook of Palliative Medicine* (eds D. Doyle, G.W.C. Hanks & N. MacDonald), pp. 257–274. Oxford Medical Publications, Oxford.

Hanks, G.W., de Conno, F, Hanna, M., McQuay, H.J., Mercadante, S., Meynadier, J., Poulain, P. & Roca i Casas, J. (1996) Morphine in cancer pain: modes of administration. Expert working group of the European Association for Palliative Care. *British Medical Journal*, 312, 823–826.

Hanna, M.H., Peat, S.J., Woodham, M. *et al.* (1990). Analgesic efficacy and pharmacokinetics of intrathecal morphine-6-glucuronide: comparison with morphine. *British Journal of Anaesth*, 64, 547–550.

Harkins, S.W., Price, D.D., Bush, F. M. & Small, R.E. (1994) Geriatric pain. In: *Textbook of Pain*, 3rd edition (eds P.D.Wall & R.Melzack), pp. 769–786. Churchill Livingstone, Edinburgh.

Harrison, A. (1991) Assessing patients' pain: identifying reasons for error. *Journal of Advanced Nursing*, 16, 1081–1025.

Hawthorn, J. (1995) *Understanding and Management of Nausea and Vomiting*. Blackwell Science, Oxford.

Hayward, J. (1975) *Information: A Prescription Against Pain.* Royal College of Nursing, London.

Heath, M.L & Thomas, V.J. (1993) *Patient-Controlled Analgesia: Confidence in Postoperative Pain Control.* Oxford University Press, Oxford.

Heaven, C.M. & Maguire, P. (1996) Training hospice nurses to elicit patient concerns. *Journal of Advanced Nursing,* **23**, 280–286.

Heidt, P.R. (1991) Helping patients to rest: clinical studies in therapeutic touch. *Holistic Nursing Practice,* **5** (4), 57–66.

Henkelman, W.J. (1994) Inadequate pain management: clinical considerations. *Nursing Management,* **25** (1), 48A–48D.

Hester, N.O., Jacox, A., Miaskowski, C. & Ferrell, B. (1992) Excerpts from guidelines for the management of pain in infants, children, and adolescents undergoing operative and medical procedures. *American Journal of Maternal and Child Health Nursing,* **17**, 146–152.

Hewitt, D. (1992) Massage with lavender oil lowered tension. *Nursing Times,* **88**, 25.

Hill, A., Niven, C.A. & Knussen, C. (1995) The role of coping in adjustment to phantom limb pain. *Pain,* **62**, 79–86.

Hillman, M., Wright, A., Rajaratnam, G., Tennant, A. & Chamberlain, M.A. (1996) Prevalence of low back pain in the community: implications for service provision in Bradford UK. *J. Epidemiol. Commun. Health,* **50**, 347–352.

Hockenberry-Eaton, M. & Sigler-Price, K. (1994) Clinical management of pain in children with cancer. *Cancer Practice,* **2**, 37–45.

Hollingworth, H. (1995) Nurses' assessment and management of pain at wound dressing changes. *Journal of Wound Care,* **4** (2), 77–83.

Holmes, S. (1991) The oral complications of specific anticancer therapy. *International Journal of Nursing Studies,* **28**, 343–360.

Horrigan, C. (1995) Massage. In: *The Nurses' Handbook of Complementary Therapies* (ed. D. Rankin-Box), pp. 125–132. Churchill Livingstone, Edinburgh.

Hoskin, P.J., Hanks, G.W., *et al.* (1989) The bioavailability and pharmacokinetics of morphine after intravenous, oral and buccal administration in healthy vounteers. *British Journal of Clinical Pharmacology,* **27**, 499–505.

Hosobuchi, Y., Adams, J.E. & Linchitz, R. (1977) Pain relief by electrical stimulation of the central gray matter in humans and its reversal by naloxone. *Science,* **197**, 183–186.

Houde, R.W., Wallenstein, S.L. & Beaver, W.T. (1965) Clinical measurement of pain. In: *Analgesics* (ed. Stevens, G.), pp. 75–122. Academic Press, New York.

Hughes, J., Smith, T.W., Kosterlitz, H.W., Fothergill, L.A., Morgan, B.A., & Morris, H.R. (1975) Identification of two related pentapeptides from the brain with potent opiate agonist activity. *Nature (Lond),* **58**, 577–579.

Hurley, A.C., Volicer, B.J., Hanrahan, P.A., Houde, S. & Volicer, L. (1992) Assessment of discomfort in advanced Altzheimer's patients. *Research in Nursing and Health,* **15**, 369–377.

Huskisson, E.C. (1983) Visual analogue scales. In: *Measurement and Assessment* (ed. R. Melzack), pp. 33–37. Raven Press, New York.

Hunt, G. & Wainwright, P. (1994) *Expanding the Role of the Nurse.* Blackwell Science, Oxford.

Husband, L. (1988) Therapeutic touch: a basis for excellence. In: *Recent Advances in Nursing: Excellence in Nursing,* pp. 25–42. Churchill Livingstone, Edinburgh.

Iadorola, M.J., Douglass, J., Civelli, O. & Naranjo, J.R. (1988). Differential activation of spinal cord dynorphin and enkephalin neurons during hyperalgesia: evidence using cDNA hybridization. *Brain Res*, 455, 205–212.

Illich, I. (1976) *Limits to Medicine: Medical Nemesis – The Expropriation of Health*. Marion Boyars, London.

Infante-Rivard, C. & Lortie, M. (1997) Relapse and short sickness absence for back pain in the six months after return to work. *Occupational Environment Med.*, 54, 328–334.

International Narcotics Control Board (1991) *Narcotic Drugs: Estimated World Requirement for 1992; Statistics for 1990*. United Nations, New York.

Inturrisi, C.E. & Hanks, G. (1993) Opioid analgesic therapy. In: *Oxford Textbook of Palliative Medicine* (eds D. Doyle, G.W.C. Hanks & N. MacDonald), Chapter 4.2.3, pp. 168–181. Oxford Medical Publications, Oxford.

Iyer, P.W., Taptich, B.J.& Bernocchi-Losey, D. (1995) *Nursing Process and Nursing Diagnosis*, 3rd edn. W.B. Saunders Company, Philadephia.

Jacobs, M.M. (1985) Low back pain. In: *Signs and Symptoms in Nursing: Interpretation and Management* (eds M. Meier Jacobs & W. Geels), pp. 152–179, J.B. Lippincott Company, Philadelphia.

Jacox, A., Carr, D.B., Payne, R. *et al.* (1994) *Management of Cancer Pain. Clinical Practice Guideline* No. 9. Agency for Health Care Policy and Research (AHCPR) Publication No. 94–0592. Rockville, MD.

Jamison, R.N., Rudy, T.E., Penzien, D.B., Mosley, T.H. Jr (1994) Cognitive-behavioural classification of chronic pain: replication and extension of empirically derived patient profiles. *Pain*, 57, 277–292.

Jayson, M.I.V. & Grennan, D.M. (1987) Clinical features of rhematoid arthritis. In: *Oxford Textbook of Medicine*, 2nd edn (eds D.J. Weatherall, J.G.G. Ledingham & D.A. Warrell), pp. 16.3–16.11. Oxford Medical Publications, Oxford.

Jensen, T.S., Krebs, B., Nielsen, J. & Rasmussen, P. (1983) Phantom limb pain, phantom pain and stump pain in amputees the first 6 months following limb amputation. *Pain*, 17, 243–256.

Jessup, B.A. & Gallegos, X. (1994) Relaxation and biofeedback. In: *Textbook of Pain* (eds P.D. Wall & R. Melzack), 3rd edn, pp. 1321–1336. Churchill Livingstone, Edinburgh.

Johnson, L.R., Mahani, B., Chan,V. & Ferrante, F.M. (1989) Modifiers of patient-controlled analgesia efficacy: I. Locus of control. *Pain*, 39, 17–22.

Johnson, M.I., Ashton, C.H. & Thompson, J.W. (1991) An in-depth study of long-term users of transcutaneous electrical nerve stimulation (TENS). Implications for clinical use of TENS. *Pain*, 44, 221–229.

Jones, A. & Doherty, M. (1995) ABC of Rheumatology: osteoarthritis. *British Medical Journal*, 310, 457–460.

Joranson, D.E. (1993) Availability of opioids for cancer pain: recent trends, assessment of system barriers, new World Health Organisation guidelines, and the risk of diversion. *Journal of Pain and Symptom Management*, 8, 353–360.

Ju, G., Hökfelt, T., Brodin, E., Fahrenkrug, J., Fischer, J.A. & Frey, P. (1987). Primary sensory neurons of the rat showing calcitonin gene-related peptide immunoreactivity and their relation to substance P-, somatostitin-, galanin-, vasoactive intestinal polypeptide- and cholecystokinin-immmunoreactive ganglion cells. *Cell and Tissue Research*, 247, 417–431.

Kaiko, R.F., Wallenstein, S.L., Rogers, A.G., Grabinski, P.Y. & Houde, R.W. (1981) Analgesic and mood effects of heroin and morphine in cancer patients with postoperative pain. *New England Journal of Medicine*, **304**, 1501–1505.

Kearney, M. (1992) Imagework in a case of intractable pain. *Palliative Medicine*, **6**, 152–157.

Kearney, M. (1996) *Mortally Wounded: Stories of Soul Pain, Death and Healing*. Marino Books, Dublin.

Keller, E. & Bzdek, V.M. (1986) Effects of therapeutic touch on tension headache pain. *Nursing Research*, **35** (2), 101–105.

Kenner, D.J. (1994) A total approach to pain management. *Australian Family Physician*, **23**, 1267–1283.

Kenyon, J. (1988) *Acupressure Techniques: A self-help guide*. VT. Rochester, Healing Arts Press.

Kodiath, M.F.& Kodiath, A. (1992) A comparative study of patients with chronic pain in India and the United States. *Clinical Nursing Research*, **1**, 278–291.

Koh, P. & Thomas, V. (1994) Patient-controlled analgesia (PCA): does time saved by PCA improve patient satisfaction with nursing care? *Journal of Advanced Nursing*, **20**, 61–70.

Kotarba, J.A. (1983) Perceptions of death, belief systems and the process of coping with chronic pain. *Social Science and Medicine*, **17** (10), 681–689.

Krieger, D. (1975) Therapeutic touch: the imprimatur of nursing. *American Journal of Nursing*, **75** (5), 784–787.

Kuhn, S., Cooke, K., Collins, M., Jones, J.M. & Mucklow, J.C. (1990) Perceptions of pain relief after surgery. *British Medical Journal*, **300**, 1687–1690.

Lamer, T.J. (1994) Symposium on Pain Management – Part II. Treatment of cancer-related pain: when orally administered medications fail. *Mayo Clinic Proceedings*, **69**, 473–480.

Lander, J. (1990) Clinical judgements in pain management. *Pain*, **42**, 15–22.

Larsen Beck, S. (1991) The therapeutic use of music for cancer-related pain. *Oncology Nursing Forum*, **18** (8), 1327–1337.

Lautenbacher, S. & Rollman, G.B. (1993) Sex differences in responsiveness to painful and non-painful stimuli are dependent upon the stimulation method. *Pain*, **53**, 255–264.

Lauritzen, M. & Olesen, J. (1984) Regional cerebral blood flow during migraine attacks by xenon-133 inhalation and emission tomography. *Brain*, **107**, 447–461.

LeResche, L. (1982) Facial behavior in pain: a study of candid photographs. *Journal of Nonverbal Behavior*, **7**, 46.

LeResche, L. & Dworkin, S.F. (1984) Facial expression accompanying pain. *Social Science and Medicine*, **19** (12), 1325–1330.

Leriche, R. (1939) *The Surgery of Pain* (translated by A. Young). Balliere, Tindall and Cox, London.

Levin, D.N., Cleeland, C.S. & Dar, R. (1985) Public attitudes towards cancer pain. *Cancer*, **56**, 2337–2339.

Levin, R., Malloy, G.B. & Hyman, R.B. (1987) Nursing management of post-operative pain: use of relaxation techniques with female cholecystectomy patients. *Journal of Advanced Nursing*, **12**, 463–472.

Levine, F.M. & De Simone, L.L. (1991) The effect of experimenter gender on pain report in male and female subjects. *Pain*, **44**, 69–72.

Ley, P. (1972) Primacy, rated importance and recall of medical information. *Journal of Health and Social Behaviour*, **13**, 311–317.

Liebeskind, J.C. & Melzack, R. (1987) The international pain foundation: meeting a need for education in pain management. *Pain*, **30**, 1–2.

Lindley, C. (1994) Overview of current development in patient-controlled analgesia. *Supportive Care in Cancer*, **2**, 319–326.

Lipowski, Z.J. (1970) Physical illness, the individual and the coping process. *Psychiatry Medicine*, **1**, 91–101.

Lipp, J. (1991) Possible mechanisms of morphine analgesia. *Clin Neuropharmacol*, **14**, 131–147.

Locsin, R.G.R.A.C. (1981) The effect of music on the pain of selected post-operative patients. *Journal of Advanced Nursing*, **6**, 19–25.

Longstreth, G.F. (1994) Irritable bowel syndrome and chronic pelvic pain. *Obstetrical Gynacological Survey*, **49** (7), 505–507.

McCaffrey, M. (1980) Understanding your patient's pain. *Nursing 80*, **10** (9), 26–31.

McCaffrey, M. (1990) Nursing approaches to nonpharmacological pain control. *International Journal of Nursing Studies*, **27** (1), 1–5.

McCaffrey, M. (1992) Pain control: barriers to the use of available information. *Cancer*, Suppl. **70** (5), 1438–1449.

McCaffrey, M., Ferrell, B., O'Neil-Page, E. & Lester, M. (1990) Nurses' knowledge of opioid analgesic drugs and psychological dependence. *Cancer Nursing*, **13** (1), 21–27.

McCaffrey, M. & Beebe, M. (1994) *Pain: Clinical Manual for Nursing Practice*. Mosby, London.

McCaffrey, M., Ferrell, B.R. & Turner, M. (1996) Ethical issues in the use of placebos in cancer pain management. *Oncology Nursing Forum*, **23**, 1587–1593.

McCaffrey, M. & Ferrell, B.R. (1997) Influence of professional vs. personal role on pain assessment and use of opioids. *Journal of Continuing Education in Nursing*, **28** (2), 69–77.

McCormack, K. (1994) Non-steroidal anti-inflammatory drugs and spinal nociceptive processing. *Pain*, **59**, 9–43.

McCracken, L., Zayfert, C. & Gross, R.T. (1992) The pain anxiety symptoms scale: development and validation of a scale to measure fear of pain. *Pain*, **50**, 67–73.

McDevitt, M.J. (1995) A(tens)tion! *Nursing*, December, 46–47.

McMahon, S. & Koltzenburg, M. (1990) The changing role of primary afferent neurones in pain. *Pain*, **43**, 269–272.

McNamara, P. (1994) *Massage for People with Cancer*. Wandsworth Cancer Support Centre, London.

McQuay, H.J. (1988) Pharmacological treatment of neuralgic and neuropathic pain. *Cancer Survey*, **7**, 141–159.

McQuay, H. & Dickenson, A.H. (1990) Implications of central nervous system plasticity for pain management. *Anaesthesia*, **45**, 101–102.

McQuay, H.J., Carroll, D. & Moore, R.A. (1988) Postoperative orthopaedic pain – the effect of opiate premedication and local anaesthetic blocks. *Pain*, **33**, 291–295.

Mackintosh, C. & Bowles, S. (1997) Evaluation of a nurse-led acute pain service.

Can clinical nurse specialists make a difference? *Journal of Advanced Nursing,* 25, 30–37.

Madeya, M. (1996) Oral complications from cancer therapy: part 2 – nursing implications for assessment and treatment. *Oncology Nursing Forum,* 23, 808–819.

Magni, G., Marchetti, M., Moreschi, C., Merskey, H. & Luchini, S.R. (1993) Chronic musculoskeletal pain and depressive symptoms in the National Health and Nutrition Examination. I. Epidemiologic follow-up study. *Pain,* 53, 163–168.

Maguire, L., Yon, J. & Miller, E. (1990) Prevention of narcotic-induced constipation. *Lancet,* 305, 1651.

Mallett, J. & Bailey, C. (1996) *The Royal Marsden NHS Trust Manual of Clinical Nursing Procedures* (eds J. Mallett and C. Bailey), 4th edn. Blackwell Science, Oxford.

Manthey, M. (1992) *The Practice of Primary Nursing.* King's Fund Centre, London.

Marcer, D., Murphy, E.J.J., Pounder, D. & Rogers, P. (1990) The pain relief clinic: how should we define success? *Journal of Intractable Pain Society of Great Britain and Ireland,* 7 (2), 9–13.

Marks, R.M. & Sacher, E.J. (1973) Undertreatment of medical inpatients with narcotic analgesia, *Annals of Internal Medicine,* 78, 173–181.

Martin, W.R., Eades, C.G., Thompson, J.A., Huppler, R.E. & Gilbert, P.E. (1976) Effects of morphine on human spinal cord and peripheral nervous activities. *Journal of Pharmacology and Experimental Therapeutics,* 197, 517–532.

Maruyama, Y., Shimoji, K., Shimizy, H. *et al.* (1980) Effects of morphine on human spinal cord and peripheral nervous activities. *Pain,* 8, 63–73.

Mason, D.J. (1981) An investigation of the influences of selected factors on nurses' inferences of patient suffering. *International Journal of Nursing Studies,* 18 (4), 251–259.

Mason, M. (1995) A fertile partnership: the role of aromatherapy in midwifery. *Aromatherapy Quarterly,* 47, 27–29.

Mather, L.E.& Mackie, J. (1983) The incidence of postoperative pain in children, *Pain,* 15, 271–282.

Maxon, H.R., Schroder, L.E., Hertzberg, V.S. *et al.* (1991) Re-186 (Sn)HEDP for treatment of pain for osseous metastases: results of a double-blind crossover comparison with placebo. *Journal of Nuclear Medicine,* 32, 1877–1881.

Mazal, S. (1978) Migraine attacks and increased platelet aggregability induced by oral contraceptives. *Australia and New Zealand Journal of Medicine,* 8, 646–648.

Meinhart, N.T. & McCaffrey, M. (1983) *Pain: A Nursing Approach to Assessment and Analysis.* Appleton-Century-Crofts, Connnecticut.

Melzack, R. (1975) The McGill Pain Questionnaire: major properties and scoring methods. *Pain,* 1, 275–299.

Melzack, R. (1984) The myth of painless childbirth. *Pain,* 19, 321–337.

Melzack, R. (1987) The short-form McGill Pain Questionnaire. *Pain,* 30, 191–197.

Melzack, R. (1990) The tragedy of needless pain. *Scientific American,* 262, 27–33.

Melzack, R. (1992) Phantom limbs. *Scientific American,* 266, 120–126.

Melzack, R., Belanger, E. & Lacroix, R. (1991) Labour pain: effects of maternal position on front and back pain. *Journal of Pain and Symptom Management*, 6, 476–480.

Melzack, R. & Katz, J. (1994) Pain measurement in persons in pain. In: *Textbook of Pain* (eds P.D. Wall & R. Melzack), 3rd edn, pp. 337–356. Churchill Livingstone, Edinburgh.

Melzack, R., Stilwell, D.M. & Fox, E.J. (1977) Trigger points and acupressure points for pain: correlations and implications. *Pain*, 3, 3–23.

Melzack, R. & Wall, P.D. (1965) Pain mechanisms – a new theory. *Science*, 150, 971–978.

Melzack, R. & Wall, P.D. (1982) *The Challenge of Pain*. Penguin Books, UK.

Menges, L.J. (1984) Pain: still an intriguing puzzle. *Social Science and Medicine*, 19 (12), 1257–1260.

Merskey, H. (1986) Classification of chronic pain. Descriptions of chronic pain syndromes and definitions. *Pain*, Suppl 3, S1–S225.

Merskey, H., Bogduk, N. (eds) (1994) *Classification of Chronic Pain Syndromes and Definitions of Pain Terms*, 2nd edn. IASP Press, Seattle, WA.

Mills, N.M. (1989) Acute pain behaviours in infants and toddlers. In: *Management of Pain, Fatigue and Nausea* (eds S. G. Funk, E.M. Tornquist, M.T. Champagne, L.A. Copp & R.A. Wise), pp. 52–59. Springer Publishing Company, New York.

Mobily, P., Herr, K., & Skemp Kelley, L. (1993) Cognitive-behavioral techniques to reduce pain:a validation study. *International Journal of Nursing Studies*, 30, 537–548.

Mobily, P., Herr, K., & Nicholson, A. (1994) Validation of cutaneous stimulation interventions for pain management. *International Journal of Nursing Studies*, 31 (6), 533–544.

Moore, S. (1997) *Understanding Pain and Its Relief in Labour*. Churchill Livingstone, Edinburgh.

Moore, S. & Holden, M. (1997) Complementary medicine for pain control in labour. In: *Understanding Pain and Its Relief in Labour* (ed. S. Moore), pp. 95–112. Churchill Livingstone, Edinburgh.

Morgan, J.P. (1985) American opiophobia: customary underutilization of opioid analgesics. *Advances in Alcoholism and Substance Abuse*, 5, 163–173.

Mount, B. (1993) Whole person care: beyond psychosocial and physical needs. *American Journal of Hospice and Palliative Care*, January/February, 28–37.

Nathan, P.W. (1988) The pathogenesis of pain. In: *Oxford Textbook of Medicine* (eds D.J. Weatherall, J.G.G. Ledingham & D.A. Warrell), 2nd edn. Oxford Medical Publications, Oxford.

Niven, C. & Gijsberg, K. (1984) Obstetric and non-obstetric factors related to pain. *Journal of Reproduction and Infant Psychology*, 2, 61–78.

Niven, N. (1989) *Health Psychology: An Introduction for Nurses and Other Health Professionals*. Churchill Livingstone, Edinburgh.

O'Brien, T. (1993) Pain. In: *The Management of Terminal Malignant Disease*, 3rd edn (eds C. Saunders & N. Sykes), pp. 33–62. Edward Arnold, London.

O'Connor, L. (1995a) Pain assessment by patients and nurses, and nurses' notes on it, in early myocardial infarction. Part 1. *Intensive and Critical Care Nursing*, 11, 183–191.

O'Connor, L. (1995b) Pain assessment by patients and nurses, and nurses' notes on it, in early myocardial infarction. Part 2. *Intensive and Critical Care Nursing*, **11**, 283–292.

Ohnhaus, E.E.& Adler, R. (1975) Methodological problems in the measurement of pain: a comparison between the verbal rating scale and the visual analogue scale. *Pain*, **1**, 379–384.

Osborne, R.J., Joel, S.P., Trew, D. & Slevin, M.L. (1986) Analgesic activity of morphine-6-glucuronide. *Lancet*, **I**, 828.

Ospipova, N.A., Novikov, G.A., Beresnev, V.A. & Loseva, N.A. (1991) Analgesic effect of tramadol in cancer patients with chronic pain: a comparsion with prolonged-action morphine sulfate. *Current Therapeutic Research*, **50**, 812–821.

Owen, H., McMillan, V. & Rogowski, D. (1990) Postoperative pain therapy: a survey of patients' expectations and their experiences. *Pain*, **41**, 303–307.

Owens, K.M. & Ehrenreich, D. (1991a) Literature review of nonpharmacologic methods for the treatment of chronic pain. *Holistic Nursing Practice*, **6** (1), 24–31.

Owens, K.M. & Ehrenreich, D. (1991b) Application of nonpharmacologic methods of managing chronic pain. *Holistic Nursing Practice*, **6** (1), 32–40.

Oxford English Dictionary (1988) 3rd edn. Oxford University Press, Oxford.

Pasternak, G.W. (1993) Pharmacological mechanisms of opioid analgesics. *Clinical Neuropharmacology*, **16**, 1–18.

Payne, R., & Gonzalez, G. (1993) Pathophysiology of pain in cancer and other terminal diseases. In: *Oxford Textbook of Palliative Medicine* (eds D. Doyle, G.W.C. Hanks & N. MacDonald), pp. 140–148. Oxford Medical Publications, Oxford.

Peate, I. (1996) How nurses make decisions regarding patient medication. *British Journal of Nursing*, **5**, 417–437.

Pellegrino, E. (1979) The anatomy of clinical judgements. In: *Clinical Judgement: A Critical Appraisal* (eds Engelhardt, Spicker & Towers), pp. 169–194. Reidal, Dordrecht.

Percival, A. (1995) *Aromatherapy: A Nurses Guide*. Amberwood Publishing, Surrey.

Plummer, J.L., Gorlay, K., Cherry, D.A. & Cousins, M.J. (1988). Long-term spinal administration of morphine in cancer and non-cancer pain: a retrospective study. *Pain*, **44**, 215–220.

Plummer J.L., Cherry, D.A., Cousins M.J., Gourlay, G.K., Onley, M.M. & Evans, K.H.A. (1991) Long-term spinal administration of morphine in cancer and non-cancer pain: a retrospective study. *Pain*, **44**, 215–220.

Pomeranz, B.H. (1994) Acupuncture in America: A commentary. *APS J*, **3**, 96–100.

Portenoy, R.K. (1990) Chronic opioid therapy in nonmalignant pain. *Journal Pain and Symptom Management*, **5** (Suppl), S46–S62.

Portenoy, R.K. (1993) Adjuvant analgesics in pain management. In: *Oxford Textbook of Palliative Medicine* (eds D. Doyle, G.W.C. Hanks & N. Mac-Donald), Chapter 4.2.5, pp. 187–203. Oxford Medical Publications, Oxford.

Portenoy, R.K., Foley, K.M. & Intrussi, C.E. (1990) The nature of opioid responsiveness and its implications for neuropathic pain: new hypotheses derived from studies of opioid infusion. *Pain*, **43**, 273–286.

Portenoy, R.K., Foley, K.M., Stulman, J. *et al.* (1991) Plasma morphine and morphine-6-glucuronide during chronic morphine therapy for cancer pain: plasma profiles, steady state concentrations for renal failure. *Pain*, **47**, 13–19.

Portenoy, R.K. & Hagen, N.A. (1990) Breakthrough pain: definition, prevalence and characteristics. *Pain*, **41**, 273–281.

Porter, J. & Jick, H. (1980) Addiction rare in patients treated with narcotics. *New England Journal of Medicine*, **302** (2), 123.

Prkachin, K.M. (1992) The consistency of facial expressions of pain: a comparison across modalities. *Pain*, **51**, 297–306.

Raiman, J. (1986) Towards understanding pain and planning for relief. *Nursing*, **11**, 411–423.

Rang, H.P., Bevan, S. & Dray, A. (1991) Chemical activation of nociceptive peripheral neurones. *British Medical Bulletin*, **47**, 534–548.

Rankin, M. (1982) Use of drugs for pain with cancer patients. *Cancer Nursing*, **5** (3), 181–190.

Rankin-Box, D. (1995) Hypnosis. In: *The Nurses' Handbook of Complementary Therapies* (ed. D. Rankin-Box), pp. 119–124. Churchill Livingstone, Edinburgh.

Rasmussen, B.K. (1993) Migraine and tension-type headache in a general population: precipitating factors, female hormones, sleep pattern and relation to lifestyle. *Pain*, **53**, 65–72.

Rawlins, M.D. (1993) Non-opioid analgesics. In: *Oxford Textbook of Palliative Medicine* (eds D. Doyle, G.W.C. Hanks & N. MacDonald), Chapter 4.2.5, pp. 187–203. Oxford Medical Publications, Oxford.

Regnard, C. (1995) Constipation. In: *Flow Diagrams in Advanced Cancer and Other Diseases* (eds C. Regnard & J. Hockley), pp. 11–13. Edward Arnold, London.

Reid, J., Ewan, C. & Lowy, E. (1991) Pilgrimage of pain: the illness experience of women with repetitive strain injury and the search for credibility. *Social Science and Medicine*, **32** (5), 601–612.

Reisine, T. & Pasternak, G. (1996) Opioid analgesics and antagonists. In: *The Pharmacological Basis of Therapeutics* (eds J.G. Hardman, L.E. Limbird, P.B. Molinoff, R.W. Ruddon & A. Goodman-Gilman), 9th edn, Chapter 23. McGraw Hill, New York.

Rimer, B., Levy, M.H., Keintz, M.K., Fox, L., Engstrom, P.F. & MacElwee, N. (1987) Enhancing cancer pain control regimens through patient education. *Patient Education and Counselling*, **10**, 267–77.

Rolling Ferrell, B. (1991) Managing pain with long-acting morphine. *Nursing*, **91**, October, 34–40.

Romano, J.M., Turner, J.A., Jensen, M.P., Friedman, L.S., Bulcroft, R.A., Hops, H. & Wright, S.F. (1995) Chronic pain in patient-spouse behavioural interactions predict patient disability. *Pain*, **63**, 353–360.

Rose, K.E. (1994) Patient isolation in chronic benign pain. *Nursing Standard*, **8** (5), 25–27.

Roth, S.A. (1988) Nonsteroidal anti-inflammatory drugs: gastropathy, deaths and medical practice. *Annals of Internal Medicine*, **109**, 353–354.

Ross, S. & Soltes, D. (1995) Heparin and haematoma: does ice make a difference? *Journal of Advanced Nursing*, **21** (3), 434–439.

Royal College of Surgeons and College of Anaesthetists. Joint Working Party (1990) *Pain After Surgery*. Report of a working party of the Commission on the Provision of Services. The Colleges, London.

Rusthoven, J.J., Ahlgren, P., Elhakim, T. *et al.* (1988) *Varicella zoster* infection in adult cancer patients: A population study. *Archives of Internal Medicine*, **148**, 1561–1566.

Ryan, E.A. (1989) The effects of musical distraction on pain in hospitalized school-aged children. In: *Management of Pain, Fatigue and Nausea* (eds S.G. Funk, E.M. Tornquist, M.T., Champagne, L.A. Copp & R.A. Wise), pp. 145–150. Springer Publishing Company, New York.

Sargent, C. (1984) Between death and shame: dimensions of pain in Bariba culture, *Social Science and Medicine*, **19**, 1299–1304.

Saunders, C. (1967) *The Management of Terminal Illness.* Hospice Medicine Publications, London.

Saunders, C. (1988) Spiritual pain. *Journal of Palliative Care*, **4** (3), 29–32.

Savage, R.A., Whitehouse, G.H. & Roberts, N. (1997) The relationship betwen magnetic resonance imaging appearance of the lumbar spine and low back pain, age and occupation in males. *European Spine Journal*, **6**, 106–14.

Sawe, J., Dhalstrom, B., Paazlow, *et al.* (1981) Morphine kinetics in cancer patients. *Clinical Pharmacology and Therapeutics*, **30**, 629–634.

Sawe, J., Svensson, J.O. & Odar-Cederlof, I. (1985) Kinetics of morphine in patients with renal failure. *Lancet*, **2**, 211 (Letter).

Scarry, E. (1985) *The Body in Pain: The Making and Unmaking of the World.* Oxford University Press, New York.

Scott, I. (1994) Effectiveness of documented assessment of postoperative pain. *British Journal of Nursing*, **3** (10), 496–501

Schechter, N.L., Allen, D.A. & Hanson, K. (1986) Status of pediatric pain control: a comparison of hospital analgesic usage in children and adults. *Pediatrics*, **77**, 11–15.

Schofield, P. (1995) Using assessment tools to help patients in pain. *Professional Nurse*, **10**, 703–706.

Seers, K. (1987) Perceptions of pain. *Nursing Times*, **83**, 37–39.

Seers, K. & Friedli, K. (1996) The patients' experience of their chronic non-malignant pain. *Journal of Advanced Nursing*, **24**, 1160–1168.

Shandor Miles, M. & Neelon, V.J. (1989) Approaches to pain in infants and children. In: *Management of Pain, Fatigue and Nausea* (eds S. G. Funk, E.M. Tornquist, M.T. Champagne, L.A. Copp & R.A. Wise), pp. 105–110. Springer Publishing Company, New York.

Simkins, P. (1989) Non-pharmacological methods of pain relief during labour. In: *Effective Care in Pregnancy and Childbirth* (eds I. Chalmers, M. Enkin, & M.J. Keirse), pp. 893–912. Oxford University Press, Oxford.

Sims, S. (1986) Slow stroke back massage for cancer patients. *Nursing Times*, **82**, 47–50.

Slater, M.A. & Good, A.B. (1991) Behavioural management of chronic pain. *Holistic Nursing Practice*, **6**, 66–75.

Sloman, R. (1995) Relaxation and the relief of cancer pain. *Nursing Clinics of North America*, **30**, 697–709.

Snelling, J. (1994) The effect of chronic pain on the family unit. *Journal of Advanced Nursing*, **19**, 543–551.

Sofaer, B. (1985) Pain management through nurse education. *Recent Advances in Nursing: Perspectives on Pain* (ed. L.A. Copp), pp. 62–74. Churchill Livingstone, Edinburgh.

Sofaer, B. (1992) *Pain: A Handbook for Nurses*, 2nd edn. Chapman & Hall, London.

Southall, D.P., Cronin, B.C., Hartmann, H., Harrison-Sewell, C. & Samuels, M.P. (1993) Invasive procedures in children receiving intensive care: preliminary report. *British Medical Journal*, 306, 1512–1513.

Spiegel, D. & Bloom, J.R. (1983a) Pain in metastatic breast cancer. *Cancer*, 52, 341–345.

Spiegel, D. & Bloom, J.R. (1983b) Group therapy and hypnosis reduce metastatic breast carcinoma pain. *Psychosomatic Medicine*, 45 (4), 333–339.

Spross, J.A. & Wolff Burke, M. (1995) Nonpharmacological management of cancer pain. In: *Cancer Pain Management*, 2nd edn (eds D.B. McGuire, C. Henke Yarbro, B.R. Ferrell), pp. 159–205. Jones & Bartlett, Boston.

Sriwatanakul, K., Kelvie, W., Lasagna, L., Calimlin, J.F., Weis, O.F. & Mehta, G. (1983) Studies with different types of visual analog scales for measurement of pain. *Clinical Phamacology and Therapeutics*, 34, 234–239.

Stacey, M.J. (1969) Free nerve endings in skeletal muscle of the cat. *Journal of Anatomy*, 105, 231–254.

Staff, P.H. (1988) Clinical considerations in referred muscle pain and tenderness – connective tissue reactions. *European Journal of Applied Physiology*, 57, 369–372.

Stanton-Hicks, M., Janig, W., Hassenbusch, S., Haddox, J.D., Boas, R. & Wilson, P. (1995) Reflex sympathetic dystrophy: changing concepts and taxonomy. *Pain*, 63, 127–133.

Stein, C., Comisel, K., Haimeri, E. *et al.* (1991) Analgesic effect of intraarticular morphine after arthroscopic knee surgery. *New England Journal of Medicine*, 325, 1123–1126.

Sternbach, R. (1987) *Mastering Pain: a Twelve-Step Regimen for Coping with Chronic Pain*. Arlington Books, London.

Stevensen, C. (1995) Aromatherapy. In: *The Nurses' Handbook of Complementary Therapies* (ed. D. Rankin-Box), pp. 51–58. Churchill Livingstone, Edinburgh.

Suhaya, R. & Kim, M. (1984) Documentation of the nursing process in critical care. In: *Classification of Nursing Diagnosis: Proceedings of the Fifth National Conference* (eds K.M. McFarland & G. McLane), pp. 166–172. C.V. Mosby, St. Louis, MO.

Sunderland, S. (1978) *Nerves and Nerve Injuries*. Churchill Livingstone, Edinburgh.

Sullivan, M.J.L., Reesor, K., Mikail, S. & Fisher, R. (1992) The treatment of depression in chronic low back pain: review and recommendations. *Pain*, 50, 5–13.

Sutters, K.A. & Miaskowski, C. (1992) The problem of pain in children with cancer: A research review. *Oncology Nursing Forum*, 19, 465–471.

Swarm, R.A., & Cousins, M.J. (1993) Anasthetic techniques for pain control. In: *Oxford Textbook of Palliative Medicine* (eds D. Doyle, G.W.C. Hanks, N. MacDonald) Chapter 4.2.6, pp. 204–221. Oxford Medical Publications, Oxford.

Swerdlow, M. (1984) Anticonvulsant drugs and chronic pain. *Clinical Neuropharmacology*, 7, 51–82.

Sykes, N.P. (1996) An investigation of the ability of oral naloxone to correct opioid-related constipation in patients with advanced cancer. *Palliative Medicine*, **10**, 135–144.

Terenius, L., & Whalstrom, A. (1973) Search for an endogeneous ligand for the opiate receptor. *Acta Physiologica Scandinavica*, **94**, 74–81.

Tesler, M.D., Savendra, M.C., Ward, J.A., Holzemer, W.L. & Wilkie, D.J. (1989) Children's words for pain. In: *Management of Pain, Fatigue and Nausea* (eds S.G. Funk, E.M. Tornquist, M.T. Champagne, L.A. Copp & R.A. Wise), pp. 60–64. Springer Publishing Company, New York.

Thomas, V. & Rose, F. (1993) Patient-controlled analgesia: a new method for old. *Journal of Advanced Nursing*, **18**, 1719–1726.

Travel, J.G. & Simmons, D.G. (1983) *Myofascial Pain and Dysfunction: The Trigger Point Manual*. Williams & Wilkins, Baltimore.

Turk, D.C. & Rudy, T.E. (1987a) IASP taxonomy of chronic pain syndromes: preliminary assessment of reliability. *Pain*, **30**, 1777–1189.

Turk, D.C. & Rudy, T.E. (1987b) Toward a comprehensive assessment of chronic pain. *Behaviour Research and Therapeutics*, **25**, 237–249.

Turk, D.C. & Rudy, T.E. (1990) The robustness of an empirically derived taxonomy of chronic pain patients. *Pain*, **43**, 27–35.

Turk, D.C. & Meichenbaum, D. (1994) A cognitive-behavioural approach to pain management. In: *Textbook of Pain* (ed. P.D. Wall & R. Melzack), 3rd edn, pp. 1337–1348. Churchill Livingstone, Edinburgh.

Turner, J., Deyo, R.A., Loeser, J.D., von Korff, M. & Fordyce, W.E. (1994) The importance of placebo effects in pain treatment and research. *Journal of the American Medical Association*, **271** (20), 1609–1614.

Twycross, R.G. (1988) The therapeutic equivalence of oral and subcutaneous/intramuscular morphine sulphate in cancer patients. *Journal of Palliative Care*, **2**, 67–68.

Twycross, R. (1994) *Pain Relief in Advanced Cancer*. Churchill Livingstone, Edinburgh.

United Kingdom Central Council for Nursing, Midwifery and Health Visiting (1992) *The Scope of Professional Practice*. UKCC, London.

United Nations (1961, amended by the 1972 Protocol) *Single Convention on Narcotic Drugs*. New York.

United Nations (1989) *Report of the International Narcotics Control Board for 1989: Demand for and Supply of Opiates for Medical and Scientific Needs*. Vienna.

Vainio, A., Ollila, J., Matikainen, E., Rosenberg, P. & Kalso, E. (1995) Driving ability in cancer patients receiving long-term morphine analgesia. *Lancet*, **346**, 667–670.

Vandenbosch, T. (1985) Chronic pain. In: *Signs and Symptoms in Nursing: Interpretation and Management* (eds M. Meier Jacobs & W. Geels), pp. 119–151. J.B. Lippincott Company, Philadelphia.

van Keuren, K. & Eland, J.A. (1997) Perioperative pain management in children. *Nursing Clinics of North America*, **32** (1), 31–44.

Vincent, C. & Lewith, G. (1994) From Beijing to Belgrade: making sense of acupuncture research. *APS J*, **3**, 89–91.

von Baeyer, C.L., Johnson, M.E. & McMillan, M.J. (1984) Consequences of nonverbal expression of pain: patient distress and observer concern. *Social Science and Medicine*, **19**, 1319–1324.

Vortherms, R., Ryan, P. & Ward, S. (1992) Knowledge of, attitudes towards, and barriers to pharmacological management of cancer pain in a statewide random sample of nurses. *Research in Nursing and Health*, 15, 459–466.

Wade, J.B., Price, D.P., Hamer, R.M., Schwartz, S.M. & Hart, R.P. (1990) An emotional component analysis of chronic pain. *Pain*, 40, 303–310.

Wainwright, P. (1985) Impact of hospital architecture on the patient in pain. In: *Recent Advances in Nursing: Perspectives on Pain* (ed. L.A. Copp), pp. 46–61. Churchill Livingstone, Edinburgh.

Wakefield, A.B. (1995) Pain: an account of nurses' talk. *Journal of Advanced Nursing*, 21, 905–910.

Walker, J.M., Davis, B.D. & Marcer, D. (1989) The nursing management of pain in the community: a theoretical framework. *Journal of Advanced Nursing*, 14, 240–247.

Walker, J., Akinsanya, J.A., Davis, B. & Marcer, D. (1990) The nursing management of elderly patients with pain in the community: study and recommendations. *Journal of Advanced Nursing*, 15, 1154–1161.

Wall, P.D. (1988) The prevention of postoperative pain. *Pain*, 33, 289–290.

Wall, P.D. & Jones, M. (1991) *Defeating Pain: The War Against a Silent Epidemic*. Plenum Press, New York.

Walsh, M. & Ford, P. (1989) *Nursing Rituals: Research and Rational Actions*. Butterworth-Heinemann, Oxford.

Ward, S. & Gatwood, J. (1994) Concerns about reporting pain and using analgesics: a comparison of persons with and without cancer. *Cancer Nursing*, 17 (3), 200–206.

Watson, C.P.N., Evans, R.J. & Watt, V.R. (1988) Post herpertic neuralgia and topical capsaicin. *Pain*, 33, 333–340.

Watson, R. (1995) *Accountability in Nursing Practice*. Chapman & Hall, London.

Weiner, J. (1994) Chronic pelvic pain. *The Practitioner*, 238, 352–357.

Weinrich, S. & Weinrich, M. (1990) The effect of massage on pain in cancer patients. *Applied Nursing Research*, 3 (4), 140–145.

Weis, O.F., Sriwatanakul, K., Alloza, J.L., Weintraub, M. & Lasagna, L. (1983) Attitudes of patients, housestaff, and nurses towards post-operative analgesic care. *Anaesthesia Analgesia*, 62, 70–74.

Weissman, D.E. & Haddox, J.D. (1989) Opioid pseudoaddiction: an iatrogenic syndrome. *Pain*, 36, 363–366.

Weissman, D.E. & Dahl, J.L. (1990) Attitudes about cancer pain: a survey of Wisconsin's first-year medical students. *Journal of Pain and Symptom Management*, 5 (6), 345–349.

Wells, N. (1990) Behavioural measurement of distress during painful medical procedures. In: *Measurement of Nursing Outcomes* Vol. 4: *Measuring Client Self-care and Coping Skills* (eds O.L. Strickland & C.F. Waltz), pp. 250–266. Springer, New York.

Whedon, M. & Ferrell, B.R. (1991) Professional and ethical considerations in the use of high-tech pain management. *Oncology Nursing Forum*, 18, 1135–1143.

White, R. (1985) Policy implications and constraints in the role of the nurse in the management of pain. *Recent Advances in Nursing: Perspectives on Pain* (ed. L.A. Copp), pp. 75–91. Churchill Livingstone, Edinburgh.

Wilkes, G.M., Ingwersen, K. & Barton Burke, M. (1994) *Oncology Nursing Drug Reference*. Jones and Bartlett Publishers, Boston.

Wilkie, D.J., Lovejoy, N., Dodd, M.J. & Tesler, M.D. (1989) Pain control behaviours of patients with cancer. In: *Management of Pain, Fatigue and Nausea* (eds S. G. Funk, E.M. Tornquist, M.T. Champagne, L.A. Copp & R.A. Wise), pp. 119–126. Springer Publishing Company, New York.

Wilkie, D.J., Holzemer, W.L., Tesler, M.D., Ward, J.A., Paul, S.M. & Savedra, M.C. (1990) Measuring pain quality: validity and reliability of children's and adolescents' pain language. *Pain*, **41**, 151–159.

Wilkie, D., Williams, A.R., Grevstad, P. & Mekwa, J. (1995) Coaching persons with lung cancer to report sensory pain. *Cancer Nursing*, **18** (1), 7–15.

Wilkinson, S. (1991) Factors which influence how nurses communicate with cancer patients. *Journal of Advanced Nursing*, **16**, 677–688.

Winningham, M.L., Nail, L.M., Barton Burke, M. *et al.* (1994) Fatigue and the cancer experience: the state of the knowledge. *Oncology Nursing Forum*, **21**, 23–34.

Woolf, C.J. (1991) Generation of acute pain: central mechanisms. *British Medical Bulletin*, **47**, 523–533.

World Health Organisation (1996) *Cancer Pain Relief*. WHO Technical Report Series. WHO, Geneva.

World Health Organisation (1994) *A Declaration on the Promotion of Patients' Rights in Europe*. WHO Regional Office for Europe, Copenhagen.

World Health Organisation (1996) *Cancer Pain Relief*, 2nd edn. WHO, Geneva.

Worsley, M.H., Macleod, A.D., Brodie, M.J., Asbury, A.J. & Clark, C. (1990) Inhaled fentanyl as a method of analgesia. *Anaesthesia*, **45**, 449–451.

Yaksh, T.L. & Malmberg, A.B. (1994) Central pharmacology of nocicieptive transmission. In: *Textbook of Pain* (eds P.D. Wall & R. Melzack), third edition. Churchill Livingstone.

Yates, P., Dewer, A. & Fentiman, B. (1995) Pain: the views of elderly people living in long term residential care settings. *Journal of Advanced Nursing*, **21**, 667–674.

Yu, X-M. & Mense, S. (1990) Response properties and descending control of rat dorsal horn neurons with deep receptive field. *Neuroscience*, **39**, 823–831.

Zborowski, M. (1979) Cultural components in responses to pain. In: *Patients, Physicians and Illness* (ed. G. Jaco), pp. 256–268. The Free Press, New York.

Zenz, M. & Willweber-Strumpf, A. (1993) Opiophobia and cancer pain in Europe. *Lancet*, **341**, 1075–1076.

Zimmerman, L., Pozehl, B., Duncan, K. *et al.* (1989) Effects of music in patients who had chronic cancer pain. *Western Journal of Nursing Research*, **11** (3), 298–309.

Zola, I.K. (1975) Culture and symptoms: an analysis of patients presenting complaints. In: *A Sociology of Medical Practice* (eds C. Cox & A. Mead), pp. 23–48. Collier Macmillan, London.

Index

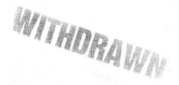
WITHDRAWN